"A passionate, sensible, and scientifica[...] enthusiastically recommend to people [...] healthy living and put their families under new management!"

—Dr. John H. Sklare
President/CEO of Inner Resource Corporation
Former Director of the Emotional Support Center at *eDiets.com*

"A book everyone should read to stem the epidemic of obesity taking over the country and to do it from a psychological, social, and spiritual perspective."

—Harold Koenig, MD, MHSc
Founder and Co-Director of the Center for Spirituality,
Theology and Health at Duke University of Medical Center
Author of *Handbook of Religion and Health* and *The Healing Power of Faith*

"Health is a family affair! And *Fat-Proof Your Family* is a refreshing and rewarding guide. It separates sense from nonsense, fact from fiction."

—Don C. Berry, PhD
President of the Institute of Religion and Health

"As a mother, my head knows what I should do for my health and that of my family. But this head knowledge isn't enough of a driving force. In *Fat-Proof Your Family*, Dr. Eaker identifies that it's your heart that drives changes toward a more healthful life. His approach is not a diet program, but a way to tap into your own path—God's specific path—for the lifelong health of you and your children."

—Karin Calloway
Editor of *Augusta Family Magazine*
Author of *Quick Cooking with Karin* and *Quick Cooking with Karin II, a Second Course*

"Our culture is failing our children. Spiritually we are minimizing God and physically we are sacrificing health for convenience and pleasure. *Fat-Proof Your Family* could not come at a better time. We the adults, the leaders, the parents need to wake up and take control of leading children and families to health once again."

—Alan Getts, MD
Pediatrician and Author of *Who Will Tell Your Children About Jesus?*

"The biblical injunction to not 'live by bread alone' certainly opens up a host of caloric choices, but it does not include user-friendly guidelines for responsible, faith-based eating habits. This dilemma is remedied by Dr. Ron Eaker who expertly integrates spiritual, medical, and psychological resources in *Fat-Proof Your Family*. Aided by an engaging writing style that exhibits both wit and wisdom, Dr. Eaker weaves practical teaching material around real-life stories. I recommend this book to both parents and professionals."

—The Rev. Dr. Sid Gates
Minister and Marriage and Family Therapist

"Dr. Eaker, in his new book *Fat-Proof Your Family*, addresses the battle that every woman and parent faces at some point in her life. It is refreshing to find that this is not just another diet book. Finally, we have a book that spells out in simple terms how to follow God's exciting plan for a life filled with health and happiness."

—Cindy Brynteson, RN
Nutrition expert and Mom

FAT PROOF YOUR FAMILY

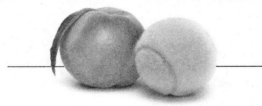

J. Ron Eaker, MD

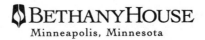

Minneapolis, Minnesota

Published by Bethany House Publishers
11400 Hampshire Avenue South
Bloomington, Minnesota 55438

Bethany House Publishers is a division of
Baker Publishing Group, Grand Rapids, Michigan.

Printed in the United States of America

ISBN-13: 978-0-7642-0413-5
ISBN-10: 0-7642-0413-0

Library of Congress Cataloging-in-Publication Data

Eaker, J. Ron.
    Fat proof your family : God's way to forming healthy habits for life / J. Ron Eaker.
        p.   cm.
    Summary: "A medical doctor addresses one of today's greatest health crises—unhealthy lifestyle choices. He provides families simple, practical, and livable plans for diet and exercise, including age-specific nutritional recommendations"—Provided by publisher.
    Includes bibliographical references.
    ISBN-13: 978-0-7642-0413-5 (pbk. : alk. paper)
    ISBN-10: 0-7642-0413-0 (pbk. : alk. paper)
    1. Nutrition—Religious aspects—Christianity. 2. Children—Nutrition—Religious aspects—Christianity. 3. Family—Nutrition—Religious aspects—Christianity. I. Title.
    RA784.E12   2007
    613.2—dc22   2007011986

God is the author of all, and to him is the glory.

To my family: Susan, Katie, and Caroline, who are there for me—mind, body, and spirit.

And to those courageous women and men who make the decision to be fit—for themselves and their children.

J. RON EAKER, MD, received his medical degree from the University of Tennessee's Center for the Health Sciences and completed his residency at the Medical College of Georgia. Practicing in ob-gyn, he has a special interest in family health and fitness. He has been listed in America's Best Doctors, is a member of numerous professional societies, and is a founding board member and vice chairman of the Institute of Religion and Health, a nonprofit group that connects the spiritual, business, and medical communities. Ron and his wife, Susan, have two daughters and live in Augusta, Georgia. When he is not doing homework with the kids, working, speaking, sleeping, or eating, he is running, having completed ten marathons including Chicago, San Francisco, and four Boston marathons.

ACKNOWLEDGMENTS

An ancient proverb states, "Whenever the student is ready, the teacher will appear." I have been blessed by many teachers along the way, even though I was not always ready to hear or understand their wisdom at the time. Nevertheless, many persisted in helping me form my ideas into a somewhat coherent proposition that is this book. People frequently ask how long it took to write *Fat-Proof Your Family*, and my honest reply is the past forty-eight years! It is a culmination of a lifetime of learning that is ongoing. I am convinced that God has a plan and purpose for each of us, and my prayer is that this book reflects a partial fulfillment of that plan.

Numerous individuals played a major role in helping this message get distributed to those meant to hear it. I am forever indebted to them for their time, knowledge, wisdom, and kindness.

Bill Jensen is a friend, agent, confidant, and advocate. He gave birth to the idea of this book, and he remains my Barnabas. Kimberly Shumate showed both kindness and foresight to connect me with Bill, and for that I am forever indebted. The folks at Bethany House Publishers—in particular Jeff Braun and Kyle Duncan, who caught the vision and made it a reality—define integrity for me. To those who took the time to read and honestly critique the original manuscript, Dr. Don Berry, Dr. Alan Getts, Cindy Brynteson, and Sid Gates, D.Min.; many thanks for making the book readable and accurate. I have been inspired by many for this book, but none as much as Covert Bailey who began the crusade for commonsense fitness years ago. Writing itself was a learned art, and Tom Bird, years ago, planted the seed that eventually grew into books, articles, and other works. My love for medicine was kindled by my dear friend and partner in medical practice, Dr. Pat Williams, who was taken from us much too soon, and my father-in-law, Dr. Bill Shirley, who still quizzes me on interesting medical cases whenever we talk. My two daughters, Katie and Caroline, are the cables that tug on Daddy's heartstrings and keep me grounded. Rooster and Bird, I love you with a passion I can't explain.

Finally, I want to thank my wife, Susan, my partner for the past fifteen years. She has been the grace when I didn't deserve it, the patience when I tried to rush it, the wisdom when I totally blew it, and the love when I prayed for it. I love you now and forever.

CONTENTS

Help, Hope, and Hold the Mayo   13

1. The Problem: Fat Is Not Where It's At!   17

2. A Beginning: Weight Control Is a
   Head Game   33

3. The Parental Mandate: Do As I Do . . . and
   As I Say   51

4. Nutrition Basics: Eat, Drink, and Be Merry   65

5. Food for the Soul: What the Bible Says About
   Healthy Eating   91

6. Children and Teens: Nutritional Specifics   111

7. Weight Loss: It's Not the Problem You
   Think It Is!   129

8. Exercise: Shake, Rattle, and Roll   149

9. Beware: Snake Oil, Scams, and Rubber Wraps   181

10. The Goal: Achieving Wholeness and Wellness
    As a Family   203

   Appendix: Exercise Techniques   209

   Additional Resources   213

   Notes   217

HELP, HOPE, AND
HOLD THE MAYO

The greatest health-care crisis in this country is not AIDS, not cancer, not heart disease, not even HMOs; it is people not making healthy lifestyle choices. Our children's generation has the potential to be the first generation in America to have a shorter lifespan than their parents. This unimaginable crisis is due to a tidal wave of obesity engulfing the country. Losing excess fat and achieving fitness are the most important, controllable, preemptive activities for health improvement in people of all ages.

One key for lasting fat loss, and what makes this book unique, is an emphasis on family. Nothing happens in a vacuum, and this includes a practical program for a healthy lifestyle. *Fat-Proof Your Family* has at its core a belief that fitness can be simple, sustainable, and practical when it is achieved within the family structure. Tools for accomplishing this include mental commitment, proper nutrition, smart exercise, emotional and spiritual well-being, and effective education. You are "fearfully and wonderfully made," and God has provided both the methods and motivation for achieving physical, emotional, and spiritual fitness.

This book is about hope—a hope that is fueled by having a goal and a plan. It will not be easy for many of you. You may be overweight and have been fighting this problem for years. You are certainly not alone. But you are just the person I want to reassure and state confidently that you can get off this roller coaster of defeat and disappointment. This book is a way to win for both you and your family. Throw away the guilt and frustration. The past doesn't dictate the future.

Several years ago Robert Fulghum wrote a wonderful bestseller called *All I Really Need to Know I Learned in Kindergarten*. In it he describes several life lessons that were tattooed on his brain from those early sandbox years. He showed how things such as sharing, making friends, and resting could be translated from the happy-go-lucky world of the preschooler to the hectic existence of the suburbanite. Its simplicity and relevance resonated in many people and awoke in them feelings of renewal.

Fat-Proof Your Family is also based on elemental building blocks that we all learned as children. For example, when it comes to food, amounts matter. In school you were given a set amount for lunch, no more, no less. What you had on your plate was enough to both fill you up and fuel you for the day's events. There were no supersize fries, Big Gulps, or double-decker cheeseburgers. You ate to fill up, not to fill out.

We learned that attitude makes a difference. "Time-out" was a pain, and we adapted quickly to the idea that our attitude could make or break the day.

We learned that Mrs. Tucker, our old-maid teacher, loved us but ruled as a benevolent dictator. It became clear early in the year that discipline was not a burden to shoulder but a tool for success. We had a glorious time, and, if we behaved, we were rewarded for our efforts.

We also learned that playing was fun. This was real playing . . . running around, chasing girls (some things never change), and climbing on jungle gyms (before the attorneys outlawed them). We didn't consciously think about it, but we learned that exercise—play—made us feel better. We enjoyed it because it was fun, a lesson many of us forgot.

We learned that rest time was necessary. We didn't like it then because we were having too much fun. But just a few minutes into the blanket-on-the-floor routine and we were "chillin'." Well, all of us but Jamie, but he forgot his medicine that day!

We learned that snacks were okay, but snacktime had rules. Little Johnny couldn't have ten Snickers bars in one day, but neither did he have to eat tofu pudding. Snacktime was fun, but with limits.

We learned that not everybody liked barbecue sandwiches. People liked different foods, and that was all right. I swapped my Twinkies for Little Debbie cakes and Isabella got some great peanut butter sandwiches for her tuna surprise.

Finally, we learned that we had a heavenly Father that loved us and created us to have fun, be healthy, and follow his ways. My favorite song from kindergarten was "This Little Light of Mine." There is no better way to get up each day than to know your light is shining as bright as God meant it to.

Fat-proofing your family is simple, practical, and livable:

🚶 Amounts matter.

🚶 We need our brain in the game.

🚶 Discipline reaps rewards.

🚶 Exercise (play) is essential.

🚶 Rest is needed.

🚶 It's not about restrictions.

🚶 Variety leads to perseverance and success.

🚶 The family that plays together, stays together.

🚶 God is our Rock and Redeemer.

These are the pillars on which this book stands. Fat-proofing is *not* about diets, fads, quick fixes, gurus, miracle cures, secret formulas, or sex, fries, and videotapes. It is not for the person who needs to lose 150 pounds. It is for average people who are overweight and concerned that their children will follow in their footsteps. It is about success, hope, and health for the entire family. It is about honoring God with your body, mind, and spirit.

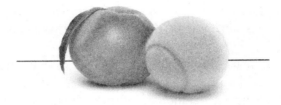

THE PROBLEM

FAT **IS NOT** WHERE IT'S AT!

Andy had not always been overweight. There was a time when he was about average, not too big, not too small. He worked well with others, so he was popular, but now he always had a feeling that people viewed him differently because of his size. He even believed that he had been passed over a couple of times when he knew he could do a job. He tried not to let the fact that he was bigger than others get in the way of enjoying life, but it was getting difficult.

Andy would come home after a hard day and snack on cookies and such, maybe have a soda, and wait on the woman in his life to get dinner ready. In the meantime he would do a little paper work, watch some TV, and diligently practice being sedentary. He would tell folks that it was his right to relax after a hard day. The last thing he wanted to do was exercise, which seemed like torture to him. Besides, when he tried sports, he noticed that he gave out before everyone else, and he was embarrassed. He was happy to just sit at home and vegetate, as he called it. He knew his weight was accumulating due largely to his inactivity, but hey, he was tired at the end of the day. At dinner, he consumed everything in front of him, whether hungry or not. He remembered being instructed years before to clean his plate, and he did what he was told. Before bed, there would be more TV and, of course, a small snack of leftover pound cake (aptly named!).When the alarm clock erupted in the morning, it was out into the day and another round of unhealthy choices.

Sound familiar? You may be surprised to discover that Andy is ten years old and represents a huge number of kids in this country.

We are raising a generation of Pillsbury Doughboys and Dough-girls, and it is our fault. The good news is, there is hope. If fault lies with us, that means we can do something about it.

My sense is that you bought this book because you are genu-inely concerned about your family's health. As a physician, but more important, as a parent, I empathize with your desire to help your family achieve its potential. You wouldn't be reading this if you weren't ready to take action and see that the people you love the most adopt and maintain a healthy lifestyle.

This book will be your coach, cheerleader, and partner in your quest for fitness. God has given you all the tools you need to win the game; your charge is to use those tools effectively. However, God never said the game will be easy. If you have struggled your entire life with excessive weight and poor fitness habits, you have a special place in my heart. You have been blamed, shamed, and named for too long, and the pain is palpable. Nevertheless, I urge you to use that pain as motivation to change. Is your present "overfat" and "under fit" situation due to decisions you make on a daily basis? Sure it is, but that is too simplistic. People are wonderfully compli-cated beings, and there are probably a hundred reasons why you have struggled with your weight over the years, but it is time to uncover a practical approach to the question, "what now?" Let go of where you have been and start to visualize where you and your family can be.

AN EPIDEMIC

Poor weight control is the number one health problem facing families today. An alarming statement in this age of AIDS, cancer, and heart disease, isn't it? And as mentioned earlier, unless we, as parents, change both our ways and our kids' habits, we may be facing the first generation of children that will die before their parents. That is an audacious assertion, so let me support this claim with some frightening statistics. As you digest this data, hold a photo of your family next to you, or at least picture your children and your spouse in your mind's eye.

- 𝕏 58 million American adults are overweight; 40 million obese; 3 million morbidly obese.

- 𝕏 60% of adults over twenty-five are overweight.

- 𝕏 78% of Americans are not meeting basic activity level recommendations.

- 𝕏 76% increase in Type 2 (adult-onset) diabetes in adults thirty to forty years old since 1990.

- 𝕏 80% of Type 2 diabetes is related to obesity.

- 𝕏 70% of cardiovascular disease is related to obesity.

- 𝕏 42% of breast and colon cancer is diagnosed among overweight individuals.

- 𝕏 30% of gall bladder surgery is related to being overweight.

- 𝕏 26% of overweight people have high blood pressure.

- 𝕏 100,000 new cases of cancer each year are due to obesity.
    Source: American Heart Association, 2004 data

Imagine two loaded 747 jetliners colliding midair and killing everyone on board: certainly a tragedy. Now imagine that happening *every single day* and you get a sense of the devastation caused by excessive fat.

You might be thinking, *Sure this stuff sounds bad, but these are adults. They can choose to harm themselves if they want to.* You're right, and indeed, that is what they are doing, but consider this:

- 𝕏 Among American children ages six to eleven, 18% of girls and 19% of boys are overweight.

🚶 Among American adolescents ages twelve to nineteen, 19% of girls and 20% of boys are overweight.[1]

That's over 13 million overweight kids. The entire population of Wyoming, Montana, Idaho, Utah, North Dakota, South Dakota, Nebraska, New Mexico, Kansas, and Alaska . . . combined!

> "Despite steady progress over most of the past century toward assuring the health of our country's children, we begin the twenty-first century with a startling setback—an epidemic of childhood obesity."
>
> *Institute of Medicine special report*, 2004

These are not numbers to be proud of! Are these your children, your family? Are we condemning them to a life of limits? Being big early in life inevitably translates into a greater risk of being big later. The likelihood of being overweight increases with age for both males and females, and overweight adolescents have a 70 percent chance of being overweight as adults. If one parent is overweight, that likelihood increases to 80 percent![2] Twenty percent (almost one-fifth) of our children over the age of six are overweight! If a quarter of our kids had AIDS, you could expect an immediate outcry. You wouldn't be able to turn on the TV without seeing some celebrity hosting a telethon. Weight control is a monumental problem—a monumental *family* problem.

HOPE SPRINGS ETERNAL

If you still have that family photo nearby, look at it closely. How are your loved ones doing now? Are they on their way to a joyful, meaningful future? What I want you to see in that photo is hope. This outlook is vital. John Maxwell, speaker and author on leadership issues, says where there is no hope in the future, there is no power in the present.

Fat-Proof Your Family is about hope—hope for a lifetime of health and wellness, hope for meaning and purpose. You see, hope is fueled by having a goal and a plan. And this book provides a plan to achieve fitness for the whole family. Hope is important because it is "the foundational quality of any change," says psychologist Alfred Adler, developer of the popular theory of personality development.

In other words, if you see any area of weight control or fitness in you or your family that needs improvement, it will require change, and that change is possible because you have hope.

I will never forget my first night in the emergency room as a medical student. I was working with the residents, taking care of a girl brought in after a suicide attempt. She was a very pretty sixteen-year-old, and I was able to get to know her a bit as she remained hospitalized for several days. After gaining her trust, I finally worked up the courage to ask her why she had tried to overdose on pills. She simply said, "I had no hope." At sixteen, she was already tired of seeing a future devoid of meaning. She felt she had nothing to live for, no hope of anything good. There is no greater feeling of desperation.

We never need to be without hope because the apostle Paul tells us, "So I pray that God, who gives you hope, will keep you happy and full of peace as you believe in him. May you overflow with hope through the power of the Holy Spirit" (Romans 15:13). Where there is love, there is hope. And what better way to love your family than to begin with the hope and expectation of health and wellness.

A FAMILY THING

Rick Warren begins his megahit, *The Purpose-Driven Life*, by saying, "It's not about you." The great thing about fat-proofing your family is that it is not only about you. This book is about being a part of a winning team—your family—and you couldn't find a better group of folks to associate with! Now, you may be saying, "Whoa, Nellie, you haven't seen my family! Our family tree is a cactus!" Nevertheless, as a parent, you have an immense impact on your family.

Imagine all the benefits that result from being fit. Imagine working *together*—supporting each other, encouraging each other, holding each other accountable—and creating bonds stronger than any World Series champion, Super Bowl victor, or winning NASCAR team. Your challenge is to embrace this responsibility with all the joy and love you can muster and lead your family into new areas of discovery.

Both my parents had a marked affect on my development, albeit in different ways. I was raised by a stepfather who was emotionally distant. He coached and encouraged sports, and I believe he tried to live vicariously through our participation. However, he was never able to connect with us on an intimate level. He was a coach, not a dad. What made this especially hard for me was that I was not particularly gifted at sports. I was the one who was picked for kickball *after* the kid in the leg cast. I was small for my age . . . or maybe just short for my height. I made up for it in effort; however, having the hand–eye coordination of a sloth, that effort often fell short— very short. (In fact, I find it ironic that I am a pretty good surgeon today.) Due to my lack of stellar, God-given ability, my stepdad would often not only be detached, but also highly critical. I found myself detesting baseball practice because I didn't want to embarrass him. To this day I break out in hives if anyone mentions grounders or fly balls. Only now can I look back and see how this influenced my desire to participate in team sports. I learned early in life that it was better not to play at all than to go for it and fail. This began a destructive pattern that haunted me until I understood its source.

Did You Know?

The best predictor of kids' long-term participation in sports is the attitude of the parents. Parents who stress the fun of simply being a part of a team or being involved in a solo activity are more likely to have children who become lifelong exercise advocates.

Fortunately, by the grace of God, I had a mother who was able to burst through the negative comments and insults and love me for the short, chubby, uncoordinated kid that I was. This literally rescued me from thinking that I was doomed in sports and in life. Through her love and encouragement, I was able to overcome my destructive thoughts and become who I was meant to be.

Fat-proofing your family can start a legacy that extends far beyond the present. That's because fitness and weight control challenges are also generational issues. Fat kids become fat adults, and fat adults tend to raise fat kids. This cycle, very much like poverty, must be broken. It is within the family where we develop our habits, both good and bad. We learn consciously or unconsciously how to shop for food, exercise (or not), handle stress, and eat. Our thoughts, imprinted at an early age, become our actions, our actions become our habits, our habits become our character, and our character determines our legacy.

THE STARTING POINT

Warren Buffett, probably one of the most successful investors of our time, once said that making money in the stock market was easy; simply buy low and sell high! Sounds easy, happens rarely. Likewise, maintaining a healthy weight and achieving fitness is based on simple principles, but the payoff is determined by the follow-through. It is persistence and discipline that creates fit families.

To prevent portliness, you must balance what you take in with what you put out. It's really that simple. In spite of the billions of dollars spent on weight loss products each year, it all comes down to this equation:

$$weight\ control = output\ (exercise/activity) - input\ (food)$$

Before going any further, we need to ask, what is a healthy weight? And how do we know if we're fit? After all, we need a standard in order to set goals.

For years we have been burdened by the "ideal weight" tables. I say burdened because they are based on a fairly arbitrary configuration. First, realize that your actual weight is not the critical consideration for assessing fitness. You are better served by understanding and embracing the idea of body mass index (BMI). Rather than looking just at body weight, BMI correlates with the amount of body fat you have. Excess body fat puts you at greater risk for health problems. Thus, BMI is the measurement of choice for many physicians and researchers studying fitness and weight control.

BMI uses a mathematical formula that takes into account both a person's height and weight. BMI equals a person's weight in kilograms divided by height in meters squared (BMI kg/m2). To simplify things, use the following table which uses inches and pounds to determine your present BMI.

Body Mass Index Table (for persons 16 years and older)

Height	Normal						Overweight					Obese										Extreme Obesity														
BMI	19	20	21	22	23	24	25	26	27	28	29	30	31	32	33	34	35	36	37	38	39	40	41	42	43	44	45	46	47	48	49	50	51	52	53	54
												Body Weight (pounds)																								
58"	91	96	100	105	110	115	119	124	129	134	138	143	148	153	158	162	167	172	177	181	186	191	196	201	205	210	215	220	224	229	234	239	244	248	253	258
59"	94	99	104	109	114	119	124	128	133	138	143	148	153	158	163	168	173	178	183	188	193	198	203	208	212	217	222	227	232	237	242	247	252	257	262	267
60"	97	102	107	112	118	123	128	133	138	143	148	153	158	163	168	174	179	184	189	194	199	204	209	215	220	225	230	235	240	245	250	255	261	266	271	276
61"	100	106	111	116	122	127	132	137	143	148	153	158	164	169	174	180	185	190	195	201	206	211	217	222	227	232	238	243	248	254	259	264	269	275	280	285
62"	104	109	115	120	126	131	136	142	147	153	158	164	169	175	180	186	191	196	202	207	213	218	224	229	235	240	246	251	256	262	267	273	278	284	289	295
63"	107	113	118	124	130	135	141	146	152	158	163	169	175	180	186	191	197	203	208	214	220	225	231	237	242	248	254	259	265	270	278	282	287	293	299	304
64"	110	116	122	128	134	140	145	151	157	163	169	174	180	186	192	197	204	209	215	221	227	232	238	244	250	256	262	267	273	279	285	291	296	302	308	314
65"	114	120	126	132	138	144	150	156	162	168	174	180	186	192	198	204	210	216	222	228	234	240	246	252	258	264	270	276	282	288	294	300	306	312	318	324
66"	118	124	130	136	142	148	155	161	167	173	179	186	192	198	204	210	216	223	229	235	241	247	253	260	266	272	278	284	291	297	303	309	315	322	328	334
67"	121	127	134	140	146	153	159	166	172	178	185	191	198	204	211	217	223	230	236	242	249	255	261	268	274	280	287	293	299	306	312	319	325	331	338	344
68"	125	131	138	144	151	158	164	171	177	184	190	197	203	210	216	223	230	236	243	249	256	262	269	276	282	289	295	302	308	315	322	328	335	341	348	354
69"	128	135	142	149	155	162	169	176	182	189	196	203	209	216	223	230	236	243	250	257	263	270	277	284	291	297	304	311	318	324	331	338	345	351	358	365
70"	132	139	146	153	160	167	174	181	188	195	202	209	216	222	229	236	243	250	257	264	271	278	285	292	299	306	313	320	327	334	341	348	355	362	369	376
71"	136	143	150	157	165	172	179	186	193	200	208	215	222	229	236	243	250	257	265	272	279	286	293	301	308	315	322	329	338	343	351	358	365	372	379	386
72"	140	147	154	162	169	177	184	191	199	206	213	221	228	235	242	250	258	265	272	279	287	294	302	309	316	324	331	338	346	353	361	368	375	383	390	397
73"	144	151	159	166	174	182	189	197	204	212	219	227	235	242	250	257	265	272	280	288	295	302	310	318	325	333	340	348	355	363	371	378	386	393	401	408
74"	148	155	163	171	179	186	194	202	210	218	225	233	241	249	256	264	272	280	287	295	303	311	319	326	334	342	350	358	365	373	381	389	396	404	412	420
75"	152	160	168	176	184	192	200	208	216	224	232	240	248	256	264	272	279	287	295	303	311	319	327	335	343	351	359	367	375	383	391	399	407	415	423	431
76"	156	164	172	180	189	197	205	213	221	230	238	246	254	263	271	279	287	295	304	312	320	328	336	344	353	361	369	377	385	394	402	410	418	426	435	443

Source: Adapted from Clinical Guidelines on the Identification, Evaluation, and Treatment of Overweight and Obesity in Adults: The Evidence Report.

To identify a goal weight using the chart, just go in reverse. Find your height—you can't change that—and then the corresponding weight for the BMI values between 18.5 and 24.9, which is considered "normal." Now, it's important to note that this BMI table is not applicable to children under sixteen. For children and teens, BMI is both age- and sex-specific. BMI values for adults do not take into account these criteria. To calculate your child's BMI, go to *www.cdc.gov*.

One variable BMI fails to consider is lean body mass. In fact, it is possible for a healthy, muscular individual with very low body fat (high lean mass) to be classified as obese using the BMI formula. If you are a trained athlete, your measured percent body fat would be a better indicator of what you should weigh. The ideal way to

BMI	Weight Status
Below 18.5	Underweight
18.5–24.9	Normal
25–29.9	Overweight
30 and above	Obese

Invest in a bathroom scale that measures BMI, which should be your standard for goal setting.

determine your healthiest weight is to have your lean body mass (muscle and bone) calculated and then add 15 percent for males and 22 percent for females. From a practical standpoint, though, most people don't have access to an accurate means to determine their lean body mass. For example, underwater tests, the gold standard in calculating lean body mass, are expensive and skinfold measurements can vary from tester to tester. Studies indicate that there is a good correlation between BMI and lean body mass; therefore, BMI is more meaningful for the average person.

Interestingly, as the following chart indicates, a person's waist size is also linked to health problems. This is because the type and location of fat we carry affects our health tremendously. Fat under the skin (subcutaneous fat) is

Did You Know?

There are reasonably priced and accurate scales that measure percent body fat. Check your pharmacy, health food store, or online . . . if you dare!

generally not too bad, whereas fat on the inside of our bodies (visceral fat) is the evil twin. Again, from a practical standpoint, in women in particular, there is a good correlation between the two fat twins, so if one is increased, the other is usually elevated.

RISK OF ASSOCIATED DISEASE ACCORDING TO BMI AND WAIST SIZE

BMI		Waist < or = 40 in. (men) or 35 in. (women)	Waist > 40 in. (men) or 35 in. (women)
18.5 or less	Underweight	—	N/A
18.5 to 24.9	Normal	—	N/A
25.0 to 29.9	Overweight	Increased	High
30.0 to 34.9	Obese	High	Very High
35.0 to 39.9	Obese	Very High	Very High
40 or greater	Extremely Obese	Extremely High	Extremely High

Source: www.consumer.gov

It is important at this point to distinguish being overweight from being obese. Obesity, in the medical community, is a distinct clinical entity that is accepted to have many causes including genetic, psychological, physiological, and social. Technically, a person is obese if he or she has a BMI greater than 30. Compared with being overweight, which is mainly treated with improved nutrition and exercise habits, obesity often involves more intense treatments.

The starting point for conquering both obesity and being overweight is not the waist, thighs, or arms. It is the brain. Studies indicate that folks tend to underestimate their weight or even fail to acknowledge whether they are overweight or obese. Recognizing and acknowledging your "real" weight status is your responsibility. Begin now by changing your paradigms about health.

First, change "me" thinking to "us" thinking. Nothing happens in a vacuum. Your health is intimately intertwined with that of your family. When you think about healthy practices—whether exercise, nutrition, or any other aspect of fat-proofing—have your family in mind. Ask yourself, "How will this affect my family? How can we achieve fitness together?" Second, understand that health is not just physical healing but a balance of mind, body, and spirit. (We'll explore this further later in the book.)

DO THE RIGHT THING

We are a culture that shirks responsibility. Blaming others, institutions, God, and life in general for our problems and misfortunes has become epidemic. Kids are masters at both skateboarding and scapegoating. Personal responsibility has become a lost virtue.

The most egregious example of this mindset was the failed lawsuit against a fast-food chain a few years ago, accusing them of making a child obese! I suspect it would have had merit if Ronald McDonald had kidnapped the young tyke and held him hostage in the basement of the local Ronald McDonald House and force-fed him Big Macs for a year. If that were the case, I would be the first to join a posse to bring in the crazed clown! But alas, the kid simply ate, and ate, and ate a mountain of fast food and became overweight. As my teenage daughter says, duh!

A recent government report chastises the food industry for its contribution to the nation's expanding waistlines. Indeed, fast-food establishments do bear

> The average child sees ten thousand TV advertisements per year.
> Source: *www.Supersizeme.com*

some responsibility; however, they are really not the problem. Limiting portion sizes and putting more low-calorie foods on the menu at restaurants may be helpful, but unless *you* change what and how much you and your family are eating, all will continue to struggle. It is not the responsibility of the restaurant owner to police your food consumption any more than it is up to the convenience store owner to determine how much gasoline you buy.

There is actually joy and satisfaction in accepting responsibility for our choices and taking back control. So how do you take control? Step number one is education. Put this book down right now and give yourself a standing ovation because you are in the process of accomplishing that objective. (Please don't do this if you are in a Starbucks or a library, as you will be asked to leave.) You have to have a basic knowledge to make wise decisions. The writer of Proverbs says, "Fear of the Lord is the beginning of knowledge. Only fools despise wisdom and discipline" (1:7).

Educating yourself and your family about fitness and nutrition must be a priority. If nutritional knowledge becomes important, then the application of this knowledge becomes real power. In this country we spend more time discussing the merits of American Idol contestants than learning which healthy foods to eat. It is this lack of balance that has generated the crisis of obesity. Take heart, though! There are massive amounts of resources to supply the facts you need to make healthy decisions. One of the purposes of this book is to distill this mountain of information into sound, simple, and practical action plans to achieve fitness.

Our education system is woefully inadequate in preparing us for real-world nutrition. Up-to-date and accurate middle school and high school courses in nutrition are as rare as compassion from the IRS. I recently reviewed my daughter's eighth-grade health text and found references to the now maligned food pyramid and an out-dated explanation of metabolism. There was no mention of the negative contribution of the fast-food industry to the childhood obesity epidemic (or the epidemic itself), the elimination of physical education in the schools, and the abundance of junk food (even at hardware stores!).

The stark reality is that good information on healthy nutritional practices is largely self-acquired. Unfortunately, most of the information our kids glean is in the form of infomercials, advertisements, and promotions disguised as news and legitimate instruction. A recent survey of American schoolchildren found that 96 percent could identify Ronald McDonald. The only fictional character with a higher rate of identification was Santa Claus.[3]

It is encouraging that some school systems are taking a more aggressive stance on childhood obesity. Recently in Arkansas, schools sent home letters to parents with their child's BMI (body mass index), telling them if their child was overweight. Arkansas has one of the highest rates of obesity in the country, and it will be interesting to see if this practice will improve their deadly standing. As is, this program is teetering on extinction due to the objections of a few parents who resent the schools labeling their kids as obese. This is a perfect illustration of parents refusing to take responsibility.

With a basic understanding of your current fitness level and BMI, it is time to initiate action. Simply apply what you learn.

Learning without doing is like sowing without reaping. The key to any person's success, whether in business or in the home, is taking action.

TAKE ACTION

Chester had always been a cautious guy. He was the kind of fellow who could walk into a room and not be noticed for ten minutes, even if there was only one other person there. He liked it that way. His motto was, "If I can avoid it, I will." He even took a job in a library so no one would talk to him, and if they did, it was in a whisper. One day Chester glanced around the bookshelves and saw the most beautiful girl he had ever seen. He was enraptured by her looks and the regal way she carried herself. He was so enamored that he almost went up to her without thinking and introduced himself . . . almost. He caught himself, and started his usual negative self-talk. "I can't speak to this girl; she would just laugh at me. Even if I did talk to her, what would I say? I doubt she has a secret desire to learn the Dewey Decimal system." So true to form, he did nothing.

Day after day this vision of loveliness would arrive in the library and Chester would drool on his card catalog, and day after day he would say nothing. After about three weeks of staring from afar, he confided in his only friend, John, about his dilemma. John was a bit of a man about town and often embarrassed Chester with his comments, but they seemed to have a true admiration for each other. John wisely explained to Chester that sitting on his bum behind the counter would never get him an introduction to this girl. Chester, as was his character, replied, "But she would probably say something back and then what would I do?" Then John spoke words of simple wisdom: "Chester, don't waste time worrying about step two, three, and four. You'll never get to them if you don't take step one." Chester eventually took that step one, and thus began my grandparents' fifty-year loving relationship. He took action—thank goodness, or I might not be here—and the results have paid off for generations.

This book is designed to motivate you to take action. It is a guide to illustrate the abundance of what God has given to each one of us and how we can use that abundance to bless our families. This book is a positive *doing* book. God lavishes gifts and graces on us all, and to make the most of those, we must be fit in mind, body, and spirit. That now becomes your challenge and charge.

In the past thirty years, Dick and Rick Hoyt have answered the call by completing more than nine hundred endurance events around the world, including more than sixty marathons and eight Ironman triathlons. John Brant writes in *Runner's World* magazine that they've run their hometown Boston Marathon twenty-four times to date. Dick and Rick are a gifted father-and-son tandem. These accomplishments alone are reason for admiration; however, Rick has severe cerebral palsy and Dick pushes him in a modified wheelchair in each and every race!

The athletic phenomenon that is known as Team Hoyt began one spring day in 1977. Rick was fifteen at the time and came home from school asking his dad if they could run a five-mile road race together to benefit a local college athlete who'd been paralyzed in an auto accident. It was a strange request considering Rick's situation. Plus, Dick was a forty-year-old non-runner. When they got to the event, organizers saw the wheelchair, the disabled son, and the middle-aged dad and gave them a look that said, "You two won't make it past the first corner." They didn't know Dick. It wasn't in his nature to quit a job he'd started. And besides, by that first corner, Rick was having too much fun. They ran the entire five miles and didn't finish last. Afterward, a wild grin lit up Rick's face. Later he tapped out on his computer: "Dad, when I'm running, it feels like I'm not handicapped."[4] From that special moment thirty years ago, when a dad decided to take action, literally millions have been inspired to be great.

It all begins with a thought! If we don't think it first, we don't do it. That's what John "The Penguin" Bingham discovered. Before his first marathon, he was an overweight, out-of-shape, middle-aged non-runner. "The miracle isn't that I finished," he says. "The miracle is that I had the courage to start."[5]

You must now find the courage to start on a path to health for you and your family. The costs of not doing so are astronomical. For you to be the best caregiver, wife, mother, husband, or father you can be, you must embrace God's desire for his children to be well. Use this book as a tool. Read it once all the way through, then go back and focus on the areas of greatest need. You will stumble; we all do. The only failure is not getting up again and doing something different, learning from your mistakes. Do it for yourself and your kids. Make fat-proofing your family a priority. Today is the first day of the rest of your bites!

—— FAT-PROOF POINTERS ——

Poor weight control is the number one health problem facing families today.

This book is about hope.

If you see any area of weight control or fitness in you or your family that needs improvement, it will involve change, and that change is possible because you have hope.

Fat-proofing your family can be a legacy that extends far beyond the present.

The solution to being overweight—the foolproof way to fat-proof your family—must encompass all aspects of family life.

Health is not just physical healing, but a balance of mind, body, and spirit.

Body mass index (BMI) is more illustrative of fitness and health than your actual weight.

Educating yourself and your family about fitness and nutrition must be a priority.

The key to any person's success—whether in business or in the home—is taking action.

Make fat-proofing your family a priority.

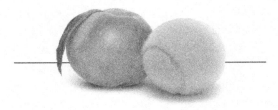

A BEGINNING

WEIGHT CONTROL IS A **HEAD** GAME

"Dad, I made a 94 on my science test!"
"Great, son. Let's get some ice cream to celebrate."

"Billy, if you behave while we shop, I'll buy you some candy."

"Samantha, you were so good with the doctor today. Here's a lollipop."

Do you recognize these conversations? I do, because at one time or another I have spoken those same words. I suspect many of you have. They sound so trivial and innocent out of context, but their impact is tremendous. Let's be honest, eating junk food tastes good, is fun, and makes for sweet rewards! It looks appealing and feels good in our mouths. It tickles the taste buds. It puts us in a good mood and, in many cases, it's even cheap. So what could be so bad with something feeling so good? I think it's a shame that God didn't make candy bars taste like broccoli. It sure would bolster our will-power.

Myth: I can't lose weight because of genetics and a "slow metabolism." **Fact:** Your biology is not your weight destiny.

This leads to the number one reason we fail in diets, teach our kids poorly, and struggle with being one of the fattest nations on earth: our brains! Don't misunderstand what I am saying. I am not saying that you are weak, lack willpower, or are a mental midget if you are overfat. I am saying that our thoughts control our actions. Remember when I said that our thoughts eventually become our legacy? That legacy, whether it is leaving millions of dollars or millions of memorable moments, begins with a thought. Whether it is eating, running, or making a shopping list, the brain generates the spark that eventually translates into action. Dr. John Sklare, author of *The Inner Diet*, says, "You can't change your weight until you change your mind."[1] If you can conquer the mental aspect of fat-proofing your family, you are well on the way to lifelong success.

FOOD FOR THE MIND

The psychology of food is a fascinating study. Many of us assume that we eat simply to fuel our bodies; however, the underlying motivation for some eating is a study in pleasure, social interaction, and cultural norms. Few of us sit down to a big Sunday dinner and think, *I know my liver is excited about this steak.* No, when we sit down to dinner, we are more concerned about why our sixteen-year-old is still at his girlfriend's than what the nutritional content of the meal is. We don't consciously think of meals as refueling; instead we tend to associate them with social interaction and habit. In fact, many of us respond to the clock for meals more than we respond to signals that our bodies need to replenish. We have become "automatized" and relatively rigid about meals.

When we dine, we respond to the texture, smell, and taste of the food along with the feeling of satisfaction that comes from the meal. Scientists are discovering physiological connections in the brain that play a role in satiety and overeating. One theory claims that overeaters consume more food because they get a magnified, pleasurable jolt from dopamine, a potent neurotransmitter or brain hormone. Ann Kelley, a researcher at the University of Wisconsin, says, "The implication is that long-term over-ingestion of foods that are highly preferred, such as fats, could have a drug-like effect on the brain."[2]

Let's be honest, most of us do get a psychological boost from eating. Even memories of pleasure can be triggered by certain foods. I will never forget the smell and the taste of the turkey and dressing my mother would make every Thanksgiving, and more important, I associate this food with a sense of peace and relaxation. In that instance, it is not just about

> Dr. John Sklare suggests three statements to memorize and incorporate into your "mental exercise" routine:
>
> - ✗ I accept some discomfort as a part of weight control.
> - ✗ Losing weight is worth the discomfort.
> - ✗ Discomfort means success.

providing protein for my muscles; it now becomes a source of positive psychological reinforcement. These can be very powerful feelings, enough so that eating can actually be an attempt for some to re-create those positive emotions. And it should! God has given us an unbelievable cornucopia of things to eat. God is about abundance and joy, and we need to celebrate that abundance . . . in moderation.

In spite of plentiful healthy choices, there are a number of radical nutrition experts whose aberrant philosophies literally equate some foods with poison. They insist, for example, that eating meat is tantamount to ingesting cancer cells. I would agree with the poison analogy if you made a rump roast with arsenic, but short of that, food is meant to be enjoyed. No one ever died by eating a piece of cheesecake. Where you court trouble is when you eat that cheesecake three times a week for twenty years.

As I stated at the outset, amounts count. Let me add another caveat: variety is healthy. There is a focus on restriction that permeates some weight loss philosophies. (In direct opposition to these programs are the fitness gurus that tell you to eat anything!) Eating a severely restricted diet is potentially as unhealthy as pizza and beer four days a week. Have the occasional southern fried steak and gravy, but just don't make it a weekly staple. Nacho cheese dip is not one of the four essential food groups, but it can be a once-a-year Super Bowl treat. Fat-proofing your family is about balance and a regular dose of uncommon sense.

The physical and psychological satisfaction from eating can lead you to try to re-create nurturing experiences through meals. We also know that food can be a very strong motivator. We as parents especially use this tool to "bribe" our children. How many of us were rewarded with a tasty piece of candy or a dessert because we were "good"? I once tried to reward my kids with an extra serving of turnips and they threatened to call the authorities! But those early reinforcements—for example, equating food, especially sugar, with being good—stick with us for a lifetime.

Are You a Chocoholic?

- Is milk chocolate how you get your dairy?

- Do you look at vanilla as a communist conspiracy?

- Do you take Nestlé's birthday off from work?

- Has an M&M never had enough time to melt in your hands?

- Is your idea of exercise kneading chocolate chip cookie dough?

- Do you think PMS stands for Pass My Sweets?

Dr. Andrew Weil, a renowned physician and health advocate, says, "I think it is fair to say that food is an important source of pleasure for most of us, and a primary source of it for some of us. For that reason any recommendations for healthy eating that diminish or eliminate the pleasure of the experience of eating are sure to fail."[3] (It is important for you to know that while I respect Dr. Weil's views on nutrition, I do not support or encourage his philosophical or religious views.) Concepts such as this combined with years of scientific research confirm that moderate weight loss is primarily a brain game.

Eric Schlosser writes a frightening exposé of the pitiful state of the American diet: "A nation's diet can be more revealing than its art or literature. On any given day in the United States about one quarter of the adult population visits a fast food restaurant. During a relatively brief period of time, the fast food industry has helped to transform not only the American diet, but also our landscape, economy, workforce, and popular culture. Fast food and its consequences have become inescapable, regardless as to whether you eat it twice a day, try to avoid it, or have never taken a single bite."[4] Schlosser goes on to make a chilling statement: "The Golden Arches are now more widely recognized than the Christian cross."[5] Junk food and poor food choices are pervasive, and we must take back control or present and future generations will suffer.

OVERFED AND OVERFAT

The reasons why someone eats too much are as varied as every person's personality. It is foolish to try to wax psychoanalytically and list all of the possible rationales. In many instances, a trained counselor can be very helpful in identifying specific issues that influence a person's particular eating habits. Some people are introspective enough to uncover subtle reasons for overeating; others can't tell you a reason, they just do it. In his book *Thin Again,* Dr. Arthur Halliday speculates that a person's excess weight is always a symptom of an underlying problem or false belief, and that permanent resolution depends on identifying and correcting the cause, whether it be physical, emotional, or spiritual. It is important to understand that this doesn't imply that there is a correlation between a person's spiritual maturity and their weight. Spiritual giants get fat, and I know some fit atheists. The point is that weight loss, fat-proofing your family, and getting fit involves a balance of mind, body, and spirit.

The most successful weight loss programs, like Weight Watchers, all recognize the enormous impact that our minds have on eating. They address that aspect with stress management, accountability, and other support techniques. Quite honestly, you only need one diet in your lifetime, the one you make up your mind to stick to!

CHANGE

You might ask, "If getting fit and losing fat is so simple, why doesn't everyone do it?" Good question! The answer is that change is hard. That's why we don't automatically alter our lifestyles even when we understand the advantages. We persist in our habits even in the midst of unhealthy behaviors that we know are killing us. Why? Because there is a perceived comfort in the known. I want you to understand that there is actually terrible danger and discomfort in the status quo. The good news is that you can win the mental battle needed to fat-proof your family. You have to decide now that this is absolutely what you must do. You have to be passionate about it.

Psychologists tell us that primarily two things motivate people to action: the avoidance of pain and the pursuit of pleasure. Think about a simple everyday task like brushing your teeth. The reason you do this is either to avoid the pain of decaying teeth and people passing out from smelling your breath, or to have the pleasure of a beautiful smile. My guess is that avoiding the pain of social isolation equates with the pleasure of a toothy grin. In fact, studies indicate that people will go to greater lengths to avoid pain than they will to seek pleasure.

> "If we don't change direction soon, we'll end up where we're going."
> —"Professor" Irwin Corey, comedian

Our behavior can be altered by changing what we believe about the pain or pleasure of a situation. Take eating as an illustration. There is a type of treatment called aversion therapy, where the practitioner associates a certain food with a highly negative physical perception. For example, every time a subject eats a cookie he gets a mild electric shock. After a while, the person learns that eating a cookie is harmful and stops doing it (unless he is a congressman; they don't seem to ever be averse to taking things). Don't misunderstand; I'm not suggesting we hook you up to a car battery every time you sit down to eat a fried green tomato. The point is that the negative reinforcement—in this case an electric shock—can be replaced by a thought. Studies indicate that an *imagined* painful consequence of eating the cookie is just as powerful as the physical stimulus.

The mind is incredibly effective at creating its own perception of reality. What does all this have to do with making healthy lifestyle choices? Simply this: By understanding the negative consequences of being overfat, having poor eating habits, and not exercising, you can form an association in your mind that inhibits the destructive behavior. You avoid the pain.

Let me emphasize that the initial step in becoming fit is getting to a place where nothing will obstruct total commitment to the idea that fitness is life sustaining. You can implant these feelings more intensely by periodically imagining opposing negative scenarios. Focus on the pain that arises from not taking action. Feel what it is like for both you and your children to suffer the ill effects of poor health. Realize that our way of life is becoming our way of death!

The entire purpose of these exercises is to stimulate a desire to change, and then maintain that course. Don't be put off by the negative nature of this approach. The consequences are too great. Throughout history people have used negative associations to change behavior, with great success. God's great prophets of the Old Testament filled the hearts and minds of the Jews with revelations of consequences if they didn't change their ways.

THE GOOD NEWS

Now realize that it is possible to alter any imagined, negative outcome for your family. Recognize that by making some simple changes (as I will outline), you can prevent those unfortunate scenarios forever. Understand and rejoice that you really can make a difference in you and in your family's lives that will last a lifetime. Experience the hope that you can take control of bad habits, reverse them, and transform lives. As a physician, I realize there are certain circumstances that contribute to poor fitness that are out of your control, such as accidents, genetic or congenital diseases, and infectious problems. But these occurrences are much less common than the controllable events.

After avoiding pain, people change behaviors most often to pursue pleasure. One source of pleasure is achieving goals. Goal setting is part of any true success formula. You have to know where you are going to be able to get there!

A pilot friend of mine once told me that when they set a bearing for a particular airport, rarely are they ever following the exact path of the flight plan. They have a goal of landing at a particular site, but reaching that goal involves numerous adjustments and recalibrations. Likewise, once you know where you are going, you have to constantly be vigilant, reevaluating your progress. A map or plan is worthless unless you know exactly where you are heading.

Often, change comes after a defining moment—an event, comment, or experience that breaks through your previously held aberrant thoughts and pushes you to adopt a new belief that aligns with your core values. Alex was fifty pounds overweight. One day his six-year-old granddaughter came up to him, gently poked his large belly, and said, "Grandma says that if you don't get skinny, you won't see me when I get married." For Alex, this was a defining moment. His desire to see his granddaughter grow up was the core value that propelled him toward a successful weight-control program.

Think of the best possible scenario for you and your family's health. Whether it is fat loss, weight maintenance, fitness, overcoming illness, or just enjoying life more, get it into your mind. What do you want for your family? Make your answers specific down to a particular weight, or a goal such as walking three miles a day, or learning a new cooking technique. The more precise the better. Remember, you have to know where you are going in order to arrive there. For example, my wife wanted to lose ten pounds. More specifically she wanted to lose ten pounds of fat. This is a subtle but exceedingly important distinction. She wrote down all the reasons she wanted to lose the weight, and wrote down all the benefits she would realize once this was achieved. She also made a list of the potential negative consequences that could occur if she didn't lose the weight. And together we set a goal of her losing ten pounds of body fat over a three-month period by exercising forty-five minutes a day and eliminating sodas. She had a very specific goal with a specific plan. She actually reached that goal sooner by making some other dietary changes, but without a specific end point, she wouldn't have had a basis for making decisions and evaluating results. She would never have been as successful if she simply said, "Gee, it would be nice to lose ten pounds." You have to train the brain before you can train the brawn.

For me, I need a specific goal for my morning runs, or I would stay in bed much more often. Knowing I am training for a certain race, for example, supplies the motivation to put one leg in front of the other on those cold mornings. I make my plan detailed, down to the miles I expect to run each day. Now keep in mind, I am just like you in that I am no world-class athlete. In my races they keep my time with a calendar, not a stopwatch! The critical factor is formulating a positive, specific, timed goal for each person in the family. Your family's health and fitness is the final objective, but you have to be very specific as to how you will get there. Write it down, pray about it, and believe in it.

Don't be afraid to ask God to help you "renew your mind" when it comes to fitness. You are a spiritual being in a physical body. Ignatius Loyola said, "Pray like everything depends on God and work like everything depends on you."

NORMAL IS . . . WHATEVER?

Part of our fitness brain-drain is due to our culture's warped sense of normal. In a society that shuns absolutes, we find ourselves floundering in a sea of confusion trying to differentiate normal from abnormal. In fact, the postmodern moral relativists will clamor that there is no abnormal. To extend their philosophy to nutrition and fitness, they would proclaim that you can eat anything you want, anytime you want. We are bombarded by the pop culture media as to what is good—never what is bad—and their proclamations become the standard for judging "normal." Slogans like "You deserve a break today" and "Grab the gusto" or "Just for the fun of it" compel us to view food as a pleasurable experience void of consequences. Needless to say,

Top Fat-Proofing *Myths*

- You burn fat only when you exercise.
- Thin is healthy.
- Dieting helps you lose weight.
- Losing weight is hard.
- The more intense the exercise program, the better.
- Skinny people eat less than overweight people.
- "Natural" means healthy.
- Kids grow out of their baby fat.
- "Low fat" is low calorie and healthy.
- Eating twice a day is better than eating six times a day.

this gives a distorted sense of reality. Food should be pleasurable, but in moderation. God has given us a plethora of choices, and he is a God of abundance, but not of gluttony! The difference is moderation.

> A survey of three hundred restaurant chefs around the country revealed that taste, looks, and customer expectations are what matter when they determine portion size. Only one in six said the calorie content was very important, and half said it didn't matter at all.
> —Barbara Rolls, Pennsylvania State University

Food is meant to be enjoyed. I have a good friend who is an absolutely amazing gourmet cook. He can spend hours in the kitchen literally creating art, and then he shares it with those lucky enough to get an invitation. If he decides to cook a dish of pork, or use mayonnaise, or even (gasp) fry something, it is a creation of passion that is meant to be enjoyed. It is a celebration of God's blessings. In fact, he often says that when he cooks he feels like he pleases God because he is doing something that God has gifted him to do. The secret—the key in a fat-proof lifestyle—is temperance. The ancient Greek ideal of everything in moderation and nothing in excess rings true when it comes to our enjoyment of food.

Moderation is a dirty word to Madison Avenue. The consumer-driven society constantly bombards our kids with a message of "supersize me," and that quickly becomes the norm for our children. If their perception of normal starts with Biggie fries, then it is no wonder that "average" portions have become grossly exaggerated. Many places don't even sell small sizes of anything, and if they do, their "small" is equivalent to yesteryear's "large"! If your mental image of normal and healthy is based on external media-driven information, you will inevitably overdo it—all the while thinking you are just being "normal." Average food portions have increased; even plate sizes in restaurants are larger to accommodate this practice.

When it comes to food, you need to think abnormally! If you do what the average American does with her diet, then you will have the problems the average American has, namely clogged arteries, huge bellies, and thunder thighs. In this instance, normal is not healthy. Don't fall into the trap of complacency by limiting yourself to "good enough" when it comes to your diet.

In many instances, the way we perceive food in this country follows the same pattern as the way we view sex. Now, before you run screaming from the room, let me explain. We are embedded in a society that is trying to destroy the definition of what constitutes normal sexual relations. The media—print, TV, movies, Internet— all proclaim the virtue of tolerance in sexual matters. Kids are growing up in a culture where acceptance of deviant and bizarre sexual behavior is viewed as a virtue. This is because children are not taught that there are absolutes. As we should know, there are right and wrong choices, and there are consequences to those choices. Again, many people's perception of normal is so distorted by what they see and hear that they have no foundation on which to base decisions about their own lives. Normal becomes what the media says is normal, and that is a very dangerous game.

This same confusion is apparent regarding nutrition. We think that it is normal to eat fast food in mass quantities. Everyone does it. Those who deviate from "normal" are labeled as kooks or extremists. Not only does our lifestyle lend itself to Big Macs and pizzas, but it also makes them ridiculously accessible. In 1968, McDonald's operated about one thousand restaurants. Today it has about thirty thousand restaurants worldwide and opens almost two thousand new ones each year.[6] A good rule of thumb for food is that if you can get it without ever leaving your car, it's probably not good for you!

We have to be vigilant about not letting the pendulum swing too far in the opposite direction. In other words, nutrition activists who proclaim all processed, commercial food is poison are just as wrong as those who eat three meals a day at McGreasy's. If your entire diet consists of tofu, bread that tastes like cardboard, and fungi casserole, you are not only being unhealthy but also very boring. You will not have massive coronary closure if you have a chicken sandwich from Burger Prince, nor will you live to a hundred by eating only tree bark.

It is time to restore some uncommon sense in the nutrition and fitness equation. If you exercise too much, it can be unhealthy. If you eat too much, it can be unhealthy. If you exercise too little, it can be unhealthy. If you eat too little of the right things, it can be unhealthy. Extremes in either direction clog up your brain and your arteries. This is a call for uncommonly practiced common sense.

A WARPED PERCEPTION

To win the mind game, you have to embrace reality. A somewhat startling revelation is that many overweight individuals don't even realize they are portly. They have fallen into the trap of a distorted sense of normal. I know on the surface that sounds ridiculous, but a recent study at the University of North Carolina showed that only 15 percent of obese individuals categorized themselves as overweight. These were common folks who met the National Institutes of Health definition of obesity (BMI greater than 30), yet they routinely underestimated their own weight. Kimberly Truesdale, one of the authors of the study, stated, "If overweight people don't identify with being overweight, then they're most likely going to ignore messages warning of health risks." She goes on to say, "People who most need to cut their weight may not realize they're in that category. Indeed, I suspect that as average waistlines grow, heavy people see themselves as having normal and presumably healthy weights."[7] To fat-proof your family you have to engage your brain early in the process, and it has to be a realistic participation.

STRESS ME OUT

You can't talk about the psychology of food without discussing the impact of stress. Stressed parents and stressed kids overeat. Again, it all starts in the brain. Until recently, psychologists reported that it was rare to diagnose kids with stress-related illnesses. That has changed. We totally stress out our kids by our expectations and lifestyles. Not long ago I read an article about a kindergartner who was seeing a counselor about aggressive behavior. The wise psychologist determined that the aberrant activity of the child was largely due to stress . . . the stress of getting into the "right" first grade! It is time to make some major changes when your six-year-old is worried about his academic career.

Whether it is a change of environment, divorce, peer pressure, busyness, or responding to a parent's anxiety, stress is magnified in the young mind. Keep ever vigilant if your child shows signs of too much stress, such as frequent physical ailments, excessive tiredness or agitation, constantly moody or depressed, falling grades, a lack of interest in previously enjoyed activities, or is unusually dependant on a parent. A recent study in the journal *Pediatrics* found that "authoritative" parents who are strict disciplinarians, with low levels of sensitivity, are far more likely to have children who are overweight by age six, perhaps because of stress.[8]

A study by Brian Wansink, PhD, a University of Illinois marketing professor, found that during stressful times, men and women craved different foods. While women tend to yearn for sweet, indulgent foods like chocolate, men usually seek hot dishes like pizza. Such preferences may reveal personality traits by creating a "synergy between person and food."

Source: *Psychology Today*, January 2001

Often, uncovering the source of the stress is a frightening and difficult task. It is like peeling back the many layers surrounding an artichoke heart. The act of introspection may create a great deal of perceived stress itself. Charles Swindoll said, "Life is 10 percent what happens to us and 90 percent how we respond to it."

STRESS RELIEF

There are myriad solutions to stress and related issues. Often, realizing that stress is a factor in poor eating behavior is the first step in overcoming its influence. There are numerous resources for stressed-out adults. But as I have proposed, fat-proofing involves the family, and it is vital to also consider ways to help the kids reduce their stress. When it comes to stressed-out kids, the following suggestions may help:

🚶 If your child has too little free time, help him change his schedule to make time for relaxation and play. Going from one organized activity to the next can be very bothersome for some children. Kids need time to be creative and imaginative, and this rarely occurs in structured settings. Make sure they have ample opportunities to simply play.

🏃 Spend time together every day, even if it is only ten or fifteen minutes. This shared time will help you better understand your child's needs and give your child the confidence sometimes needed to tell a parent she wants to quit an activity. Don't fall into the trap of "quality" time. There is no substitute for face-to-face interaction.

🏃 Parents may want to examine their own schedules. Often a parent's hectic schedule will cause a child to be stressed or nervous about the things she is doing. Stress is contagious. A stressed-out parent often leads to a stressed-out child.

🏃 Discuss your child with his pediatrician. Occasionally, when a more serious problem is present, the pediatrician may recommend additional outside help. Don't dismiss unusual behavior as just a phase. Identifying stress in kids early allows for a swifter resolution of the problem.[9]

Stress Management for Kids

Children who have experienced stress for some time need extra patience and reassurance. They might respond to a combination of the following:

🏃 Physical contact—hugging helps children relax and builds self-esteem.

🏃 Listening—ask children how they feel.

🏃 Encouragement—help children find something they are good at and tell them how proud you are of them.

🏃 Honesty and openness—talk to and encourage children to express their feelings openly.

🏃 Security—try to be consistent.

🏃 Physical exercise—exercise helps burn off stressful feelings.

🏃 Humor—help children see the funny side of things.

🏃 Quiet—allow for quiet time.

🏃 Balanced diet—encourage children to eat a healthy, varied diet.

Source: David Elkind, in *The Hurried Child*

We struggle with all manner of life stressors and toils. Life is tough. Yet, inevitably, two characteristics of successful survivors stand out. First, they have a strong spiritual faith: a firm moral and ethical foundation upon which to make decisions and deal with adversity. Second, they have supportive family and friends who provide comfort and advice. There is no substitute for the "presence" of family and community.

Take inventory of the major stressors in your life. Pray, listen, and act. Ask God to provide you with assistance. In prayer, you are not reminding God that you need help in identifying your sources of stress. He is already aware of this. You are reminding yourself that you need God's help in discernment. Jesus teaches, "So don't worry about tomorrow, for tomorrow will bring its own worries. Today's trouble is enough for today" (Matthew 6:34).

View your family's concerns from an eternal perspective and immediately they become less monumental. Scripture provides that eternal perspective, and this worldview is available to us if we reframe our thinking. Much of our anxiety arises from self-imposed shoulds, coulds, and woulds.

> One effective tool for stress management is to stop focusing on your own problems and help someone else. This is a powerful way of shifting the emphasis from "Woe is me" to "Whoa, it's me!"

I have a wonderful patient and friend who suffered a stroke a few years back. She is severely limited in her speech and physical abilities, yet she has a spirit that soars. Before her stroke, she was a talented pianist who served as her church's organist for years. She can no longer play, but she still is an amazing witness. Every time I see Juanita she gets a big smile on her face and says, "Pray much, no worry!" I have never received better advice.

Paul says in Romans, "Do not conform any longer to the pattern of this world, but be transformed by the renewing of your mind" (12:2 NIV). So how do we literally change our minds about our family's health? How do we renew our minds with the goal of staying that way? If fat-proofing your family is a mind game, then it is time to let the games begin!

GET MOTIVATED

The process of motivating and committing oneself to action has been the subject of human study since Eve convinced Adam to eat fruit. How do we renew our minds to set us on the track for change? First, you must understand your roles. That is plural because in most families people play various roles. Why is this important in the context of mentally preparing yourself to fat-proof your family? It gives you a foundation upon which decisions can be made. It makes it clear the necessity for making healthy lifestyle decisions.

Let me give you an example. If one of your roles in the family is to be primarily responsible for cooking, it becomes your charge to learn as much as you can about preparing healthy meals and then execute the menus. If your child thinks a home-cooked meal is eating at a cafeteria instead of Burger King, you might have a problem.

Renewing the mind—motivating you to action from a scriptural basis—should involve two areas: prayer and Bible study. Philippians 4:6–7 states, "Don't worry about anything; instead, pray about everything. Tell God what you need, and thank him for all he has done. If you do this, you will experience God's peace, which is far more wonderful than the human mind can understand. His peace will guard your hearts and minds as you live in Christ Jesus." Prayer leads to transformed minds and hearts, and that in turn leads to action. Continuing on in Philippians, Paul writes, "Fix your thoughts on what is true and honorable and right. Think about things that are pure and lovely and admirable. Think about things that are excellent and worthy of praise" (4:8). This is a great example of the guidance that is readily available in Scripture if we will study and glean from its pages.

Finally, you must believe that health and wellness can be a part of your family's present and future. You can be the one who inspires your spouse and your children to see beyond the present and get a mental image of what they can be. Many overweight people think of themselves as always being "big" people. They are myopic in how they see their place in the world. Some would claim that "accepting the way you are" is a realistic and healthy psychological state of mind. If I had hypertension, and "accepted" and was "at peace" with my hypertension but did nothing to control it, then I would not be doing myself any favors. Pop psychology has made it hip to not place value judgments on people's actions and situations. That approach is hogwash! There is a difference between right and wrong, good and bad, and moral relativism has no place in our beliefs. There is no shame or intolerance in understanding the necessity of absolutes. C. S. Lewis writes, "Any attempt to create an ethic without God is doomed to failure, and without God there is no absolute standard for good and evil."[10] One absolute is that fit folks are well on the way to a balance of mind, body, and spirit.

—— FAT-PROOF POINTERS ——

Fitness, weight loss, and wellness are first and foremost a mind game.

Getting our brain in the game involves avoiding pain and seeking pleasure.

Being overweight and unfit is painful.

Being fit is pleasurable.

A passionate commitment to lifelong health only comes by deciding that you want to avoid the pain and enjoy the pleasure.

Set specific goals for each family member (with their input) and write them down.

You can be the motivator for yourself and your family.

If you can't make the mental commitment, don't waste your time with the latest diet *du jour*.

The battle of the bulge is won between the ears.

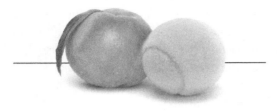

THE PARENTAL MANDATE

DO AS I DO . . . **AND** AS I SAY

Randall came home tired from another long day at work on the assembly line. He had worked at the local Ford plant for fifteen years and was an avid fisherman, spending most of his free time with a rod and reel. This evening Johnny, his nine-year-old son, was waiting for him by the door. He hugged his dad and said, "Daddy, can I ask you something?"

"Sure, buddy, what is it?"

"Daddy, how much money do you make at the plant, like how much in an hour?"

Randall was a bit taken back and gruffly said, "That's not any concern of yours." Feeling somewhat embarrassed to discuss this, he walked off.

Johnny persisted and pleaded, "Aw, Daddy, come on, I just want to know how much you get for an hour."

Knowing his son was stubborn, he reluctantly submitted and

told him that he made around twenty dollars an hour.

Johnny looked up at his dad and asked, "Then, can I borrow ten dollars?" Now Randall was getting angry. He retorted, "If the only reason you wanted to know how much money I made was to squeeze me for something to buy some dumb toy, then just turn around and go straight to your room and think about how selfish that is. I am busting my rear end to provide for this family and I don't have the time or patience for these games."

Johnny quietly went up to his room without uttering a word. After a while Randall calmed down, and as usual after he blew up, began feeling guilty. Maybe his son needed something important after all. In fact, he didn't remember him ever asking for money before. He went up to Johnny's room, gently cracked the door, and stuck in his head. "Son, are you still awake?" he asked.

"Yes, Daddy."

"Son, I think I was kind of harsh a few minutes ago and I'm sorry. Here's the ten dollars you asked for."

Johnny shot up in the bed with a big grin on his face. He then reached under his pillow and pulled out some dollar bills and began counting. Randall, seeing that the boy already had some money, started to get angry again. He asked, "If you've already got the money, why do you need more?"

Johnny replied, "'Cuz I didn't have enough, but now I do. Daddy, I have twenty dollars now. Can you play with me for an hour?"

Children spell love T-I-M-E. Fat-proofing your family takes time. There is no greater charge for a parent than taking the time to teach your children to make healthy lifestyle choices. Reading this book, setting goals, and educating yourself on the fat-proof lifestyle are good places to start; however, you literally can't sit on this information. If you don't act on this knowledge, the power is gone, and so is your influence. There is no more powerful instrument of persuasion than modeling. "The most important health-care delivery system in the world is the mother," says Dr. Richard Klausner, the former director of the National Cancer Institute.

One of my favorite child-rearing authors is John Rosemond. He captured the importance of time in parenting with the following reflections.

> *There are no quick fixes in child rearing. You can get a meal in a minute at McDonald's, but there's no such thing as McParenting. I have often had the feeling, during conversations with parents who are seeking solutions to problems they're having with their children, that they think psychologists can perform feats of time-defying magic.*
>
> *A typical encounter: The parents describe the problem, I propose a means of solving it, and the parents counter with, "Oh, we tried that already, and it didn't work." It is almost inevitable that upon further investigation I discover that "it" didn't work simply because the parents didn't work at it. They believe in McParenting.*[1]

You can't McParent fitness and health. It is a time-consuming participation sport. Conventional wisdom and the parenting experts are revising their positions on the *quality* versus *quantity* debate. For years permissive parenting manuals used quality time propaganda to justify their own absence. In this country, if you feel guilty for doing something poorly, you just reinvent the psychology to accommodate the improper behavior and conveniently erase your guilt. We see examples of this in the debate over defining marriage, sexual mores, drug use, and about any activity that rejects the notion of absolute right and wrong. If we see the world in a postmodern, secular humanist framework, then all we have to do to clear our conscience is alter the morality with psychobabble. People justify amoral behavior from a need to counter feelings of shame and guilt. These same people should realize that guilt arises from foundational beliefs in right and wrong—even if they don't consciously acknowledge it. People have feelings of guilt because they realize at some level they are acting badly. As a culture, we need to spend less time justifying our actions and more time acting justly.

There are absolutes in morals, ethics, and religious beliefs. Without foundational beliefs our families crumble into chaos; there is no basis for decision making. Interestingly, even professed atheists agree that things such as incest and murder are bad. Yet when you question them on how they determine whether something is good or bad, inevitably they have to admit there is some standard somewhere from which a determination is made. If there is something deemed as bad, there has to be something good to provide the logical contrast. If there is a standard to judge good and bad, then, again logically, there has to be a source of that standard. That source has to transcend culture and time since we have already seen the fallacy of relative values, and simple observation shows that a particular culture cannot set such standards. God is the only source that transcends time and place to provide the absolutes from which all determinations of good and bad, right and wrong, can be made.

One of those absolutes is that parenting is not a correspondence course!

A DEVOTION TO FAMILY

Rick Husband was a devout man of God. He was also an extraordinary astronaut, father, and husband. He was chosen to be the commander of the 107th space shuttle mission and was accompanied by six other men and women. Space shuttle Columbia was launched on January 16, 2003. Before he left, Rick had videotaped sixteen devotions for his two children, Laura and Matthew, one for each day he was to be gone. Eight minutes before eight o'clock on the final morning, gauges started to lose readings in Columbia's left wing and left landing gear brake system. All vehicle data was lost when the space shuttle broke up over north-central Texas. Evelyn, Rick's wife, said that the healing from the loss was helped by the lasting memory of both the devotions Rick created and the memories made at the dinner table when he was there. She said, "We all desire to give our children treasures of the heart. One of the simplest ways is to tell the stories of how God works in our own lives. My husband and I began telling our stories at dinnertime. 'Have I ever told you about the time that God. . . ?'

> "The concept of personal responsibility is not tenable in children. No child chooses to be obese. Furthermore, young children are not responsible for food choices at home or at school, and it can hardly be said that preschool children, in whom obesity is rampant, are in a position to accept personal responsibility."
>
> —Robert Lustig, MD,
> USCF Children's Hospital

or 'Have I told you about what God is doing with. . . ?' By this we can leave stories of faith as treasures for tomorrow."[2]

EATING TOGETHER

The dinner table is a powerful tool for binding families together. It is like the gathering places of old where the business of the day, both joys and concerns, were voiced. Unfortunately our culture has largely lost the custom of family dining. Increasingly, families are spending less face time together, and this is having a devastating effect on the family structure. In today's sound-bite, hurry-up, wolf-it-down society, the family table is more likely used for homework projects than meals. Sharing a meal breeds conversation even when talking to one another is normally strained. It keeps you abreast of what is happening in your kid's life. On the other hand, not sitting down to meals leads to disassociation and poor communication. This was highlighted by a fascinating study by Dr. Elena Poveda, published in the *Journal of Epidemiology and Community Health*. She looked at 259 kids ages fourteen to twenty who lived at home and compared the number of meals, on average, they ate with the family during a week. She then broke these groups into a study group of kids diagnosed with anxiety and depression disorders and those who were similar in circumstances (family income, two parents at home, etc.) yet had no mental disturbances. She found a higher percentage of the depressed kids ate many fewer meals with the family than the control group. Dr. Poveda concluded, "Sharing daily meals with the family constitutes a union ritual that promotes adolescent mental health."[3]

According to a Columbia University survey, teenagers who eat with their families at least five times a week are more likely to get

Table Talk Tips

⚓ Ask everyone to share their favorite part or biggest challenge of the day.

⚓ Plan the next day's dinner together.

⚓ Share your own childhood memories.

⚓ Discuss an activity the family can do together.

⚓ Talk with your children about a book they are reading or a movie they have seen.

Source: *www.Family.gov*

better grades in school and much less likely to have substance abuse problems. Researchers found that the teens were 42 percent less likely to drink alcohol, 59 percent less likely to smoke cigarettes, and 66 percent less likely to try marijuana. The survey also found that frequent family dinners were associated with better school performance, with teens who had structured, regular family meals 40 percent more likely to get A's and B's.

"At a time when kids are under a lot of stress for a lot of different reasons, having that regular mealtime that they can count on, that their parents are there for support—that can be very helpful," says David Elkind, a professor of child development at Tufts University in Massachusetts.[4]

START MEALS TOGETHER "EARLY"

The medical community is now validating what the Bible taught generations ago: family matters. Children usually aren't shopping for food or making decisions about what to eat for dinner, says Dr. Christopher Bolling, medical director for the Cincinnati Children's Medical Center. "You're not going to have any success if you approach just the child because the child doesn't have complete regulation over the environment. You have to go after the family."[5] The earlier you start healthy eating practices the better. At a recent seminar, one parent was complaining about her teen not eating well, and another brave parent responded, "You have to start young. A five-year-old doesn't know he has choices!"

The message is clear; the family that eats together has a better shot at developing quality relationships. "A meal is about civilizing children," says Robin Fox, an anthropologist who teaches at Rutgers University. "It's about teaching them to be a member of their culture." I want to take that further in the context of our discussion. The family that eats well stays well. It seems like such a simple concept because it is! Both science and common sense supports that regular family meals promote communication, caring, and healthy habits. This is a prime opportunity to teach kids and spouses about the joy of simple, well-chosen, practical dietary habits. Remember, variety is good, amounts count, and it is about abundance and not restrictions.

Beginning and Maintaining a Family Meal Ritual

⚹ Set a specific time for dinner. If that is not realistic due to schedules, start where you are. Find a time, whether it is Sunday after church or Saturday at breakfast, and make it a priority to have a meal together.

⚹ Don't discuss problems at meals . . . initially. Let the conversation find that path if it is natural. Keep things positive.

⚹ Involve all family members. Start by asking specifics about the day's events, or even getting comments on news items of interest.

⚹ Have consistent seating. People like consistency—even kids!—and having "my" seat at dinner implies you are important and expected to be there.

⚹ Minimize distractions. No TV, radio, Internet, or cartwheels!

⚹ Clearly define expected end-of-meal rituals. "Can I be excused?" or "Great dinner, Mom. You are a gift from God that just keeps on giving." (Yeah, dream on!)

⚹ When it's all said and done, don't be so rigid that meals become a stress-filled battleground.

LIVE IT

When I choose a race to run, I like to make it a "destination" marathon. With so many races, it is easy to find one in a spot that has a variety of other things to see and do. One of the main reasons I take the time and expense to cart my entire family to marathons is to have them experience the ambiance. I want them to see Dad not just talking about fitness, but living it. I want them to grow up understanding that exercise is normal, even expected. This sets the benchmark as to what kids understand as normal. They learn by modeling. They consciously see and incorporate in their sponge-like minds the idea that exercise is fun.

I remember the last time we were in Boston for a marathon. We spent the afternoon before the race in the runner's expo, a huge gathering of competitors and exhibitors with products and services specific to runners. After wandering around and surveying this mass of fit folks, my youngest daughter looked up at me and said, "Daddy, is everyone always this skinny and happy?" This was a marvelous teachable moment. She got it! It validated my precept that just being there allowed her to associate fitness with joy. The message was subtle but lasting. (By the way, my wife thought most of the people looked anorectic, so I prohibited her from talking to the kids the rest of the day.)

Did You Know?

The Boston Marathon was the first marathon in America. Eighteen runners started at the shout of "Go" for that race in 1897.

Certainly you don't have to run marathons to exert an impact on your family. In fact, simply going out for a daily walk sends a message to everyone. If you make it a priority, exercise will begin to be viewed as an important, necessary activity. As a parent, you have to set the example. Make it a fun family activity. Talk to your kids about your exercise plans; better yet, include them in the planning and participation. Go for a walk, shoot hoops, ride bikes, or throw the Frisbee (there may be college scholarships in this someday). If your children see you as a sedentary poster child for couch potatoes, they will inevitably incorporate that in their behavior, because they see that as normal. Now, some kids are just rebellious. They see whatever mom and dad are doing, and promptly and deliberately do the opposite. It's called establishing their independence (some call it adolescent brain damage!). However, I am convinced—and studies support—that early exposure to proper modeling behavior imprints in kids the desire to be active.

You can tell children ad nauseum to be active and exercise, but if they don't see you participating, the impact will be minimal. Again, I want to stress that this doesn't mean you have to become a semipro basketball player or a world-class gymnast. It means walking, going to aerobics, playing catch, kicking a ball, in-line skating, weight lifting, riding a bike, jogging on a treadmill—just doing something to improve your fitness consistently and persistently.

IT'S YOUR CALL

Writer Marcelene Cox described parenting as that state of being better chaperoned than you were before marriage. Kids are always there and always watching. Because of this, there is no one more responsible for fat-proofing your family than you. A simple experiment will adequately illustrate this conclusion. Go over to the refrigerator, open the door, and peer inside. Close the fridge door and wander to a cupboard and gaze in. What did you see? Whatever was there, in both places, was there because you bought it and brought it home. Now, if your ten-year-old routinely does the shopping or if you have just purchased a fully stocked new house, you are off the hook; this little exercise has no meaning for you. Still, chances are good that you and your spouse are 100 percent responsible for the food content of your home. Your family is only going to eat what is there and available. The majority of what your family eats is directly or indirectly influenced by *your* choices. You set the tone. The Talmud, the Jewish book of wisdom, states, "When you teach your son, you teach your son's son."

BECAUSE THE BIBLE TELLS ME SO

We have a biblical mandate to teach our children about how to avoid unhealthy habits and how to live joyfully. The apostle Paul wrote, "Don't make your children angry by the way you treat them. Rather, bring them up with the discipline and instruction approved by the Lord" (Ephesians 6:4). Proverbs 22:6 tells us, "Teach your children to choose the right path, and when they are older, they will remain upon it." This verse from Proverbs is especially convicting in how it applies to health and wellness. A laudable goal of parenting is to raise children who learn to be independent, happy, productive, and pleasurable to God. Parents, whether together or separate, must take responsibility for being living examples of healthy lifestyles. It's not brain surgery; well, maybe in a way it is. You have to "cut out" the unrealistic images, the lack of knowledge, the poor motivation, and the self-doubt and embrace a new mental attitude—an attitude that will promote positive change for generations to come.

A LEGACY WORTH LEAVING

One of the greatest legacies any parent can bestow on a child is this gift of knowing how to make healthy lifestyle choices. And the gift is presented by words and deeds. Josh Billings, a humorist in Mark Twain's day, said, "To bring up a child in the way he should go, travel that way yourself once in a while." There is incredible wisdom in that simple quote. It highlights the fact that we, as parents, can't get away with poor health habits and expect our kids to not to follow suit. This is the "I do as I see you do" generation, a legacy that is reflected in studies like those done at the Cooper Institute, the premiere center for the study of aerobic exercise and health. In 2005, they published research that concluded, "Adolescent body fatness is moderately related to selected adult cardiovascular risk factors."[6] In simple terms, fat kids become adults that are more prone to heart attacks and strokes. Indeed, what your kids do now will influence them for a lifetime.

> "Don't be afraid to take a big step when one is indicated. You can't cross a chasm in two small steps."
> —David Lloyd George, British statesman

Sandra was sick and tired of being sick and tired. She was both forty years old and forty pounds overweight. She, her husband, and her three children were the typical carpool family, going here and there, often waving to each other as they passed on the highway to the next activity. After a checkup discovered Sandra's cholesterol to be dangerously high, she decided to take action. At first it was simple things like walking around a track while her daughter was at soccer or changing from whole milk to skim milk. After two months, Sandra's friends and family were noticing a change. She had lost fifteen pounds and had more energy. But to Sandra, the greatest benefit was the comments of her kids: "Gee, Mom, you look great" or "How far did you go today?" The motivation to continue on this healthy path was cemented one day when she overheard her teenager on the phone saying, "Mom was working out this morning before I got up. You know, I hope I can do all that stuff when I'm her age." The seeds were planted and the family will reap the harvest.

SERVANT LEADERS

Parents must be servant leaders when it comes to fat-proofing their family. A servant leader is often a description devoted to husbands; however, I feel this model applies to both parents as it relates to children. The biblical mandate for this type of interaction stems from Luke's gospel. "But among you, those who are the greatest should take the lowest rank, and the leader should be like a servant. Normally the master sits at the table and is served by his servants. But not here! For I am your servant" (22:26–27).

Jesus emphasized that the primary motivation for all effective leaders, husbands, wives, CEOs, presidents, and parents should be the desire to serve. This is not to imply that you become a doormat for your preschooler. (It is ironic that you spend the first two years of your child's life teaching him to walk and talk and the next sixteen telling him to sit down and be quiet!) This is also not to insinuate that we have to live up to the example of Jesus . . . we can't. But we can learn from his teachings and life. What this means is that you recognize that a primary function of a parent is to meet the basic needs of the child and eventually, hopefully, prayerfully teach them to meet their own needs. One of those basic needs is choosing health-promoting lifestyles.

The bottom line is that servant leaders are leaders who put other people's needs, aspirations, and interests above their own. Replace *servant leader* with *parent* in the previous sentence and I think you can grasp the similarity. Many management experts and family therapists have embraced the concept of servant leadership as an effective tool for parenting.

How do we as parents become servant leaders in our family? Ken Blanchard, author and management consultant, writes in his book *Lead Like Jesus* (Thomas Nelson) that there are two aspects of leadership. The first is understanding that leading is a "transformational journey." By that he means this form of leadership doesn't happen overnight. It is a process and a commitment that involves many layers.

Blanchard says the second aspect of leadership (parenting, in our case) is to master what he calls the four domains of leadership:

heart, head, hands, and habit. The first domain, heart, is characterized by asking the question, "Am I a servant leader (parent) or a
self-serving leader?" In other words, what is your motivation? Are
you teaching your kids to be fit solely to live vicariously through
their athletic achievements, or are you hoping to instill lifelong
health habits that will benefit them and their children?

The next domain, head, is looking at the beliefs and theories
you have about parenting. Do you believe in modeling behavior or
only "do as I say, not as I do"? You have a parenting style whether
you know it or not. Take time to think about how your children
learn, and decide if your parenting style is facilitating that. For
example, many kids learn best by physically doing an activity—as
opposed to others who learn best by hearing or reading about something. If your child is a doer, then taking her for a walk or encouraging her to accompany you on a bike ride will register best in her
mind. If your child is more auditory in her learning style, telling her
stories of great athletes may be more motivating than running a mile
with her. You have to seek and understand a child's learning style to
be able to effectively meet his or her needs.

The third domain is hands. This means taking action. All the
knowledge in the world is useless unless it is acted upon. Change
how you cook, walk that extra mile on the treadmill, stop snacking
in the evening. These are all actions that get you closer to your goal
of healthy living. A recent survey said that over 80 percent of people
who buy self-help tapes never listen to them all the way through.
Health clubs will tell you that over 45 percent of the memberships
they sell are not utilized more than a month after they are purchased. You have to take action as a leader and as a parent. Taking
action with the kids can be as simple as transporting them to a local
park. Once they are there, they will make their own fun through
continual motion. But if they never get there, that opportunity is
lost.

The final domain, according to Blanchard, is habits. This is the
daily commitment as a parent to serve rather than to be served. If
you can't make the daily mental commitment to living a healthy
lifestyle, don't waste your money on the latest diet book or weight
loss pill. It won't work! As a parent, you have to get up every day

and mentally say to yourself, *I am going to do at least one thing today to help my family get fit, and I will make wise, healthy choices.*

It is absolutely imperative to fixate in your consciousness your role as the primary influence on your child's beliefs about health and wellness, and begin today to adopt a parenting style that encourages good nutrition, exercise, and spiritual health. Make it a simple, fun, and continual part of your life and the dividends will pay off for years. You love your kids and want the best for them. We all do. Make that love real by instituting positive food choices, living an active lifestyle, and loving God with your heart, mind, and soul.

—— FAT-PROOF POINTERS ——

Fat-proofing your family takes time.

Good health decisions have good consequences and poor health decisions lead to poor outcomes.

The dinner table is a powerful tool for binding families together.

Teenagers who eat with their families at least five times a week are more likely to get better grades in school and much less likely to have substance abuse problems.

"Family" matters when it comes to fit versus fat.

There is no one more responsible for fat-proofing your family than you.

You have a biblical mandate to teach your children about how to avoid unhealthy habits and how to live joyfully.

Parents must be servant leaders when it comes to fat-proofing the family.

Make love real by instituting positive food choices, living an active lifestyle, and loving God with your heart, mind, and soul.

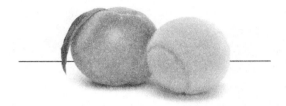

NUTRITION BASICS

EAT, DRINK, **AND** BE MERRY

"Hey, Mom, what's for dinner?" Alex shouted his familiar cry from the hall.

"I hope it's not tuna surprise . . . again," added his smart-alecky sister Emily.

"Just for that I'm going to cook your dad's old socks and T-shirt!" Angela retorted.

"Yum, yum," chimed in the youngest daughter, Rachel.

"Really, Mom, what are we eating tonight?" pleaded Alex as he reached the kitchen. "I'm starved."

Angela paused before replying. "Let's see, we all got up this morning at six-thirty and had breakfast, then I took you to school and I went to work. I got off work and picked you all up from school and took you to baseball and Emily to gymnastics. Rachel didn't have cheerleading practice today, so she went with me to get the taillight fixed on the car, then I went back and picked you both up at your activities. We came home and you guys started home-work and I started the wash. It's now six o'clock and your dad will be home anytime. Now, I ask you, when do you think I would have had time to prepare a Martha Stewart meal?"

"Mom, get a grip. I'll settle for a hot dog!" said Emily.

"Hey, pizza delivery sounds good to me," chimed in Alex.

Rachel couldn't resist adding her two cents' worth. "Mom, chill. I could live on banana pudding and Gatorade."

"You guys win; get me the phone book," said an exasperated Angela.

HUNGRY FOR . . . KNOWLEDGE?

Proper nutrition is the cornerstone of almost all our health issues. Every activity we undertake is possible only because we fuel our cells with the stuff that makes us work. Weight control, cancer, energy level, immune system, depression, and heart disease, to mention only a few, are dramatically affected by what we eat, when we eat, and how we prepare what we eat. Despite this, as a culture, we tend to devalue nutrition; either we associate it with health fanatics or we ignore it altogether. In fact, you may only think of nutrition when you see some silly infomercial touting the latest wonder food. There is a tremendous "ostrich potential" when it comes to nutrition: just bury our heads in the sand and no harm will come to us.

This paucity of education and lack of perceived value is devastating to our family's health. Alok Bhargava, a University of Houston economics professor writing in the *British Journal of Nutrition*, says, "Nutrition education is still relatively cheap in comparison with some of the treatments that overweight people may need, such as the cost of treating diabetes. I think policy makers need to consider the cost of educating the public versus treating obesity-related illness—anything less is a waste of resources."[1]

The lack of emphasis on nutrition even extends to how we train doctors in this country. Dr. Andrew Weil writes, "The poor advice about diet and health that people get far too often when they ask physicians, nurses, registered dieticians, and other representatives of the health-care establishment for help reflects the dearth of good nutritional education in our professional schools."[2]

In four years of medical school, I received ten hours of formal training in nutrition. Granted, I went to medical school before electricity (just kidding), and thankfully it does seem that strides are being made to update medical training. In 1976, approximately one out of every five medical schools in the United States required a separate course in nutrition. By 1991, one out of every four medical schools required a nutrition course.[3] Most U.S. medical schools now report that nutrition is integrated into other courses in the curriculum, and two-thirds of all schools provide an *elective* course in nutrition—one students can skip if they desire. The fact remains that in our hurry-up, fast-food, genetically altered world, healthy nutrition often continues to take a backseat. The result of this ignorance is that our collective backseats are expanding at a remarkable rate.

Societal expectations create an illusion that "normal" people eat what they have in front of them. Messages some of us have swallowed include "Don't be weird, everyone eats junk!" and "The quicker, the less effort, the better." Junk food is more pervasive than telemarketers at mealtime, and just as toxic. You can stroll into virtually any retail outlet and be faced with a feast of candy bars and snacks. Even electronic stores and bookstores sell junk food at their counters. The emphasis is obviously on economics, not health, with our children as popular targets. The marketing departments of food manufacturers understand that if they make their product easy to get, relatively inexpensive, and attractive to kids, they will make a fortune. "It's the largest market there is," says James McNeal, a professor of marketing at Texas A&M and an authority on marketing to children. "Kids 4 to 12 spend on their own wants and needs about $30 billion a year. But their influence on what their parents spend is $600 billion. That's blue sky." McNeal points out that marketing "tie-ins" are everywhere, including SpongeBob SquarePants Popsicles, Oreo

> Eighty-five percent of leading food brands that target kids in TV ads also have games and other material on the Internet. The sites promote snacks, cereal, fast food, sugary drinks, and candy. More than five hundred "advergames," such as Hershey's Syrup Squirt, Lifesavers Boardwalk Bowling, and M&Ms Trivia, are offered on seventy-seven Web sites.
>
> Source: Kaiser Family Foundation study, 2006

Cookie preschool counting books, Keebler Scooby-Doo cookies, and even a Play-Doh Lunchables playset.[4]

For those of you who are sick of hearing about nutrition, prepare to get sicker. I know that doesn't sound good coming from a physician, but the information in this chapter is crucial and will serve as your guide in making healthy decisions. Here you will find knowledge, and when knowledge is acted upon there is power. Where there is power, there is hope for change, because the power of action is what fuels the engine of results.

Next to exercise, no single activity influences your health more than what you eat . . . or don't eat. So pay attention! Your life depends on it. T. Colin Campbell writes in his revolutionary book, *The China Study,* "The provocative results of my four decades of biomedical research, including the findings from a twenty-seven-year laboratory program, prove that eating right can save your life."[5]

When it comes to nutrition, you must understand the language. It is exceedingly frustrating to walk into my car mechanic's shop and have him start orating about the manifold exhaust valve on top of the carburetor's coupled gear shaft accelerator. He may as well be speaking Swahili. He and I don't communicate well because I don't know the vocabulary. I am as dumb walking out of his shop as I was walking into it. Come to think of it, that may be his intention! But it should not be the plan for your family's health. Take the time to learn some basic vocabulary so you can truly understand and apply these concepts. If you don't, you will be a less than effective role model to your children. It is an unfortunate reality that we cannot depend on the traditional educational system or the conventional media to provide accurate and timely nutrition information.

You can be the teacher your kids so desperately need by learning a few basic facts. Don't feel bad, though, if you don't master the various nutrition terms . . . for now. I am constantly reviewing this material and reminding myself of its importance, so refer to the following pages frequently.

LABELS

Everything we eat for fuel can be broken down into six categories: water, carbohydrates, fats, proteins, vitamins, and minerals.

(Everything but Twinkies . . . and God only knows what's in those!) These distinctions are even more relevant today because of the ubiquitous food labels that adorn almost every item in grocery stores. Look at any label and you will see the nutritional content separated into these categories. For some, these labels are a blessing, and for others, a curse. My kids hate it when I pull out their box of Honey Nut Fruit Granola Cheese Doodles and quote the figures on the label. "Well, my, my . . . this only has 898 fat calories per serving, and a serving is two doodles!"

Some people think nutrition labels are just more information than they need to know. These are the denial dudes and dudettes. It is their belief that if you don't read the label, you don't get the calories. Unfortunately, this is a case of what you don't know *will* hurt you. The point is, these labels are important, and they are the first practical step in under-standing the content of your food. But if you don't know what the terms mean, it is as if the label is in ancient Sanskrit.

> ### Deciphering "Fat" Claims
>
> ⊀ "Reduced fat" means that a product has 25% less fat than the same regular brand.
>
> ⊀ "Light" means that the product has 50% less fat than the same regular product.
>
> ⊀ "Low fat" means a product has less than 3 grams of fat per serving.

Almost every packaged food is garnished with a "Nutrition Facts" label that spells out the protein, fat (polyunsaturated, saturated, and trans), carbohydrate, sodium, and cholesterol content (see sample label that follows). It also lists total calories and serving size. Take special note of the term "percent daily value" (% DV). This is an oft ignored piece of information, yet it is very important in determining how a particular item fits into the overall scheme of your daily consumption. Understanding the percent daily values can help you choose foods that are high in good nutrients and low in non-nutrients. A 5% DV or less means the food item has little of that particular nutrient; a 20% DV or more means the food has a lot of that nutrient. So for nutrients such as fat, saturated fat, trans fat, cholesterol, or sodium—nutrients we tend to overconsume—look for foods with a low % DV. Conversely, seek out foods with a high % DV for "good things" including dietary fiber, vitamin A, vitamin C, calcium, and iron.

Nutrition Facts

Serving Size 1 cup (228g)
Servings Per Container 2

Amount Per Serving

Calories 250	Calories from Fat 110

	% Daily Value*
Total Fat 12g	18%
Saturated Fat 3g	15%
Trans Fat 1.5g	
Cholesterol 30mg	10%
Sodium 470mg	20%
Total Carbohydrate 31g	10%
Dietary Fiber 0g	0%
Sugars 5g	
Protein 5g	

Vitamin A	4%
Vitamin C	2%
Calcium	20%
Iron	4%

* Percent Daily Values are based on a 2,000 calorie diet. Your Daily Values may be higher or lower depending on your calorie needs:

	Calories:	2,000	2,500
Total Fat	Less than	65g	80g
Sat Fat	Less than	20g	25g
Cholesterol	Less than	300mg	300mg
Sodium	Less than	2,400mg	2,400mg
Total Carbohydrate		300g	375g
Dietary Fiber		25g	30g

One thing to consider is that the % DV is based on a 2,000-calorie diet, which is the average energy needs for a seven- to ten-year-old; therefore, your older children and teens will likely need more than 100% DV. (For specific calorie needs for kids, see chart on page 136.) Also remember that the percent daily values are listed for a single serving, so if you eat two servings, you should double the daily value.

Make it a habit to become intimately involved with food labels (sounds risqué, doesn't it?). It is vital to have a working knowledge of these terms so that you can then use that knowledge in a practical and beneficial way. Remember that knowledge is not power, it is the *application* of knowledge that is true power. For you to be a power "full" eater, you have to know this stuff.

PROTEINS

Proteins are the building blocks for muscles, tissues, and organs. Proteins also serve double-duty as hormones (those dastardly critters), enzymes, and antibodies. Antibodies are the hit men for the immune system, seeking out and destroying invading germs. Proteins are like the body, frame, and engine of a car; they are the stuff we are made of.

Proteins consist of even smaller building blocks called amino acids. The number and type of the amino acids in a protein determines the size, shape, and length of the molecule.

In terms of practical human fuel, proteins can be divided into two categories: complete and incomplete proteins. This doesn't refer to their psychological makeup ("You complete me!"), but rather to the amino acid content of the protein. Complete proteins contain all of the nine essential amino acids that the body can't make on its own. They are called essential amino acids because it is essential that we get them from a food source. Incomplete proteins contain some, but not all, of the essential amino acids. Most animal proteins are complete proteins whereas most plant proteins are incomplete.

> **Did You Know?**
>
> ✗ Eggs contain the highest quality food protein known.
>
> ✗ While it is customary to throw rice at weddings in many countries, French brides break an egg on the threshold of their new home before stepping in, for luck and healthy babies.
>
> ✗ White-shelled eggs are produced by hens with white feathers and white earlobes.
>
> ✗ Brown-shelled eggs are produced by hens with red feathers and red earlobes.
>
> ✗ There is no difference in nutrition between white and brown eggs.

This is not a value judgment; just because a protein is incomplete does not mean it is bad or useless—quite the contrary. By eating a variety of incomplete protein sources, such as many different plants, you can easily obtain all of the essential amino acids your body craves.

It is a myth that total vegetarians suffer from protein deficiencies. Veggie lovers can get plenty of protein and all of the essential amino acids by eating a variety of plants (soy, beans, chickpeas, etc.). In fact, many studies now indicate that plant protein is generally healthier than animal protein. To take that a step further, Colin Campbell writes, "Animal protein intake was convincingly associated in the China Study with the prevalence of cancer in families."[6] He goes on to suggest that a diet that obtains most of its protein from plant-based sources may even prevent cancers and heart disease.

The evidence is overwhelming that a vegetarian-based diet is a healthy approach to eating, and that applies to the consumption of protein. Be aware, however, that moderation is more important than restriction. We should celebrate the diversity of foods God has provided. Eating lean meat on occasion is just as healthy as eating broccoli on occasion, but you wouldn't want to make either a part of every meal. Once again, the foundation upon which to build healthy, sustainable eating habits is everything good in moderation, nothing in excess.

PROTEIN CONTENT OF SELECTED ANIMAL FOODS

Animal Protein	Protein Content
Eggs (1 medium)	6 grams
Milk (1 glass)	6.3 grams
Fish (cod fillets 100g or 3.5 ounces)	21 grams
Cheese, cheddar (100g or 3.5 ounces)	25 grams
Roast beef (100g or 3.5 ounces)	28 grams
Roast chicken (100g or 3.5 ounces)	25 grams

Lean meat and dairy are good sources of protein.

PROTEIN CONTENT OF SELECTED VEGAN FOODS

Vegetable Protein	Protein Content
Soybeans, cooked (1 cup)	29 grams
Veggie dog (1 link)	8–26 grams
Veggie burger (1 patty)	5–24 grams
Lentils, cooked (1 cup)	18 grams
Tofu, firm (4 ounces)	8–15 grams
Chickpeas, cooked (1 cup)	15 grams

Black-eyed peas, cooked (1 cup)	13 grams
Soymilk, commercial, plain (1 cup)	3–10 grams
Bagel (1 medium)	9 grams
Peanut butter (2 Tbsp.)	8 grams
Spaghetti, cooked (1 cup)	7 grams
Broccoli, cooked (1 cup)	5 grams
Whole wheat bread (2 slices)	5 grams
Potato (1 medium)	4 grams

Vegetarians can get plenty of protein! One cup of soybeans has as much protein as a chicken breast.

Source: USDA Nutrient Database for Standard Reference, 1998

YOUR PROTEIN NEEDS

A simple tool for calculating your average protein need for a day is:

Ideal body weight (in pounds) $\times$ 0.36 = recommended protein intake (grams)

This is just a guideline. You have to take into consideration your body type, exercise level, and age. For example, athletes, adolescents, and pregnant or breast-feeding women need slightly more protein in their diets to meet the extra needs of their bodies. Daily protein requirements are hotly debated by various weight loss gurus. Some claim high-protein diets are remarkably healthy, whereas others state too much protein accelerates the aging process. I believe the truth lies in-between.

Because of its many uses, a deficiency in protein can lead to a variety of problems. A true protein deficiency is relatively rare in Western developed countries. However, with the advent of fad diets, more and more people are suffering severe nutritional problems. The most common cause of protein deficiency is simply poor nutritional choices.

It is apparent that certain medical conditions, such as mal-absorption of nutrients from the gastrointestinal (GI) tract, surgical therapies, and gastric bypass, can result in protein deficiencies. Complications that may result from a lack of quality protein in the diet include fatigue, insulin resistance, hair loss, hair color changes, loss of muscle mass, low body temperature, and immune and hormone imbalances.

On the opposite end of the spectrum, too much protein can also be harmful. If misused, the high-protein, low-carbohydrate diets that are periodically popular can lead to a predisposition for autoimmune diseases, renal and liver damage, and bone loss. This is especially serious for menopausal women at risk for osteoporosis. To be fair, these problems are rare even in people who maintain these restricted diets over an extended period. The good news is that few people actually can maintain these restricted diets over a long time!

CARBOHYDRATES

Carbohydrates are our major source of energy. I realize that some of you may have a hard time believing anything beneficial can come from carbohydrates because of the low-carb craze; however, carbohydrates are vital fuel for our bodies. A carbohydrate-free diet is a death wish! Carbohydrates come in two basic forms: complex and simple. Simple sugars are easily identified by their taste: sweet. Complex carbs, such as potatoes, are pleasant to the taste buds, but not sweet. Complex carbohydrates also contain dietary fiber, an important component of a healthy diet. If proteins are the body of the car, carbohydrates are the gas.

Simple sugars are commonly found in fruits, milk products, and ordinary table sugar. Complex carbohydrates, also known as starches, are found in cereals, grains, and some root vegetables.

COMMON SOURCES OF CARBOHYDRATES

Whole grain cereals	Candy	Beans	Peas
Table sugar	Cakes	Biscuits (plain)	Jam
Bran	Honey	Barley	Cornmeal
High-fiber breakfast cereals	Oats	Shredded wheat	Pasta

Check out the incredible variety!

Carbohydrates are energy powerhouses. However, overindulgence in carbohydrates (or anything, for that matter) is not healthy. Anything you consume that is not used immediately by the body is either eliminated or stored for later use. For example, if you spend most of your day watching *The Jerry Springer Show* or *The Young and the Worthless,* the energy you consume in the form of food, so anxious to be utilized, is put away for a rainy day. That generally is not a bad thing except that it is put away on your hips, thighs, and rear end. Understand that it is not necessarily the carbohydrates that create those lovely rolls of cellulite; it is the unused calories, regardless of the source.

Carbohydrates get blamed for the obesity problem largely because they make up an excessive amount of calories in the average diet. If you ate 90 percent protein, but still consumed 5,000 calories a day and did no exercise, you can bet your ham hocks you

> **Myth:** Low-carbohydrate diets result in long-term weight loss.
> **Fact:** Low-carb diets may help you lose an initial few pounds (mostly fluid) but are unhealthy in the long term. These diets often lack key nutrients found in carbohydrate foods.

would be super sized! For optimal health, cut the total calories, not necessarily only the carbohydrates.

Excess carbohydrate is initially broken down in the body and stored as either glycogen (a quick energy source for muscles and the brain) or fat (a good energy source but one that is not as readily available). The bottom line—and some of our bottom lines are bigger than others!—is that carbohydrates are perfectly healthy in moderation. Many of the carbohydrate-rich foods contain additional vitamins and nutrients that make up a healthy diet. Carbohydrates should be your major energy source, but every good thing can be overdone. The diversity of carbohydrates is immense and so is their utility. They contain amazing substances such as antioxidants that act like little gobblers circulating in your body chewing up tiny nasties.

Certain types of carbohydrates are better choices if you or your kids want to lose or maintain weight. The secret to choosing the best carbs to eat is in their ranking on the glycemic index (GI). The glycemic index is a measurement of the effect a food has on your blood sugar level. Some high-sugar foods such as maple syrup, honey, and candy, as well as foods that are "starchy" such as carrots, potatoes, and cereals, are rated high on the glycemic index. Other foods, especially foods high in fiber such as whole-grain rye bread and bran cereal, are rated low on the glycemic index because they do not produce such a rapid rise in blood sugar and insulin. When you eat high-glycemic foods you will experience a substantial rise in your blood sugar level. This, in turn, raises your blood insulin level. Insulin is responsible for transporting glucose into muscle and storage cells for metabolism.

> Balance is the key. A recent study from Harvard says those who eat a low-carb diet and get most of their protein and fat from vegetables rather than animal sources cut their heart disease risk by an average of 30 percent.
> Source: *New England Journal of Medicine,* November 2006

Some researchers postulate that spikes in your insulin level can contribute to fat deposition. The higher and more prolonged the insulin reaction, the more likely your body is to convert sugar to fat. There are some holes in this theory; however, there is enough evidence to try to limit your intake of carbohydrates with a high-glycemic index rating. In addition, a rapid rise in insulin levels can drive the blood sugar too low, which results in hypoglycemic symptoms such as shakiness, foggy thinking, fatigue, and anxiety. A recent review of the current scientific literature showed that fifteen out of sixteen published studies found that the consumption of low-glycemic index foods delayed the return of hunger, decreased subsequent food intake, and increased satiety (feeling full) when compared to high-glycemic index foods.[7] In addition, the results of several small short-term trials (one to four months) suggest that low-glycemic diets result in significantly more weight loss or fat loss than high-glycemic diets.[8] There are no long-term studies to see if this trend continues over the years, but the information looks promising. Simply stated, look for low-glycemic carbohydrates and make them the staples of your daily intake. Can you safely eat high-glycemic carbohydrates? Of course! Just do it in moderation.

Almost all commonly consumed foods have been tested to determine their standing on the glycemic index. There are a number of online sites, including *www.glycemicindex.com*, that give precise information on about any food you can imagine. They also give parameters as to what is high and what is low. I encourage you to explore this information and use it to make wise choices.

COMMON FOODS GLYCEMIC INDEX (GI) (Low is < 55, High is > 70)

Food	GI	Serving Size	Net Carbs
Peanuts	14	4 oz (113g)	15
Bean sprouts	25	1 cup (104g)	4
Grapefruit	25	½ large (166g)	11
Pizza	30	2 slices (260g)	42
Low-fat yogurt	33	1 cup (245g)	47
Apples	38	1 medium (138g)	16
Spaghetti	42	1 cup (140g)	38
Carrots	47	1 large (72g)	5
Oranges	48	1 medium (131g)	12
Bananas	52	1 large (136g)	27
Potato chips	54	4 oz (114g)	55
Snickers bar	55	1 bar (113g)	64
Brown rice	55	1 cup (195g)	42
Honey	55	1 tbsp (21g)	17
Oatmeal	58	1 cup (234g)	21
Ice cream	61	1 cup (72g)	16
Macaroni and cheese	64	1 serving (166g)	47
Raisins	64	1 small box (43g)	32
White rice	64	1 cup (186g)	52

Food	GI	Serving Size	Net Carbs
Sugar (sucrose)	68	1 tbsp (12g)	12
White bread	70	1 slice (30g)	14
Watermelon	72	1 cup (154g)	11
Popcorn	72	2 cups (16g)	10
Baked potato	85	1 medium (173g)	33
Glucose	100	(50g)	50

Remember, low GI (< 55) is good, high (> 70) is bad.
Source: *www.nutritiondata.com*

FATS

Do you know what you call someone on a no-fat diet? Dead! Fats are essential; it is just that we tend to get too much of a good thing. Fats, also known as lipids, act as a magnificently concentrated source of energy. In addition, they help the body utilize vitamins, keep the skin healthy, and help in the secretion of hormones. To continue with my car–nutrient illustration, fats are the oil that lubricates the engine and also keeps the exterior shiny.

A helpful method for categorizing fats is to divide them into saturated and unsaturated. Saturated fats are solid at room temperature and come chiefly from animal sources. Some common examples are butter, lard, meat fat, and solid shortening. These fats tend to raise the level of cholesterol, a fat-like substance in the blood. Unsaturated fats, which include monounsaturated fats and polyunsaturated fats, are liquid at room temperature and generally come from plant oils such as olive, peanut, corn, cottonseed, sunflower, safflower, and soybean. These fats tend to lower the level of bad cholesterol in the blood.

For most of us, reducing our saturated fat intake is crucial. As noted, fats are separated into saturated and unsaturated depending on differences in their chemical structure. The practical distinction is that saturated fat consumption has been linked to the development of heart disease, while unsaturated fat is less likely to cause this problem. You must have some fat in your diet for the body to function properly. The problem arises when we overdo it. There are no magic bullets, no wonder foods, and likewise there are few completely awful foods.

The most effective way to decrease the saturated fat in your diet is to eat less meat, red meat in particular. This not only decreases your total calorie and fat intake, but has numerous other benefits. For example, a 1987 study showed a marked improvement of PMS symptoms in women with a low saturated fat diet.[9]

Did You Know?

Trans fat is coming under fire from fast food, of all places. Just recently KFC, McDonald's, Wendy's, Kraft, Con-Agra, Frito-Lay, and even Disney theme parks have cut way back or stopped using trans fats in their products.

Researchers are also looking into possible links between dietary fat, elevated estrogen levels, and cancer. In one study, women who consumed 25 percent of their calories from fat experienced a decrease in serum estrogen levels as opposed to women who ate 40 percent calories from fats.[10] This may partially explain why low-fat, high-fiber diets seem to reduce your risk of breast cancer.

Excessive fat intake is associated with a multitude of health problems. Atherosclerotic heart disease, the leading killer of men and women over fifty, is intimately linked to dietary saturated fat intake. High LDL cholesterol (the bad kind), diabetes, stroke, and obesity are all increased by a diet high in saturated and trans fats.

Trans fats (also known as trans fatty acids) are particularly sinister characters in the fat family. They have been shown to be indelibly linked to cardiovascular problems such as heart attacks and strokes. The data linking these substances to diseases is so convincing that the FDA has recently mandated that labels now must list the trans-fat content of foods. Trans fats are found in foods such as vegetable shortening, some margarines, crackers, candies, baked goods, cookies, snack foods, fried foods, salad dressings, and many processed foods. When you see "hydrogenated" or "partially hydrogenated" oils in an ingredient list, the food contains trans fats.

Nuts and seeds contain a high percentage of fat; however, the fat calories are largely derived from polyunsaturated essential fatty acids. These fats are not only less harmful, but as the name implies, they are also essential for proper body functioning. Dr. Ronald Norris, noted researcher, says that polyunsaturated fats should constitute about 15 percent of your total daily caloric intake.[11]

Type of Fat	Main Source	State at Room Temperature	Effect on Cholesterol Levels
Monounsaturated	olives; olive oil, canola oil, peanut oil; cashews, almonds, peanuts, and most other nuts; avocados	Liquid	Lowers LDL (the bad one); raises HDL (the good one)
Polyunsaturated	corn, soybean, safflower, and cottonseed oils; fish	Liquid	Lowers LDL; raises HDL
Saturated	whole milk, butter, cheese, and ice cream; red meat; chocolate; coconut oil	Solid	Raises both LDL and HDL
Trans	most margarine; shortening; partially hydrogenated vegetable oil; deep-fried chips; many fast foods; commercial baked goods	Solid or semi-solid	Raises both LDL and HDL

Try to limit fat intake to mono and polyunsaturated fats, the first two categories.
Source: Harvard School of Public Health

The public gets besieged by a lot of conflicting information about fat consumption. Regardless of the hype, always remember this: There is no question that a low-fat diet contributes to your overall health. As Covert Bailey says, "You've got to release the grease, baby!" The problem with low-fat diets (and many low-fat products) is that the maxim of balance is forgotten and sugar is increased to "make up" for the decreased fat. Low-fat or no-fat does not necessarily mean low-calorie! So don't get hoodwinked into thinking you are doing something good for yourself and your family. In reality, we can usually only get less fat and sugar by just reducing the portions of those foods that are high in these substances.

The take-home message on dietary fat is to moderate your intake and be careful of the type of fat you consume. Saturated fat and trans fat are the pipe cloggers. Minimize these and live longer and better.

Dr. Rex Russell summarizes a healthy approach to fat consumption in his marvelous book *What the Bible Says About Healthy Living*. "Enjoy any fat found in a created food: nuts, seeds, fruits, vegetables, and legumes. We can enjoy pure butter and any unrefined liquid oils that have been protected from air, light, heat, and chemicals. They have proven to be better for us than chemically extracted oils. The best oils for cooking are virgin olive oil and butter. Even fat found in the marbled flesh of 'clean' animals, birds, or fish is healthful. What should be avoided? Processed oils, hormone or antibiotic laden animals, cover fat or suet, margarine, and meat eating animals."[12] God, the Great Designer, knew what was best for his creation long before the invention of cholesterol measuring devices or cardiac stress tests!

VITAMINS

Vitamins are any of several organic substances that usually are separated into water-soluble (the B-vitamins, vitamin C) and fat-soluble (vitamins A, D, E, K) groups. They are essential for our normal health and growth. Vitamins are widely diverse in chemical structure and function. They are distinct from carbohydrates, fats, and proteins in function, as well as in the quantities in which we require them. Vitamins act as necessary components in many physiological pathways. If a vitamin is absent from our diet or is not properly absorbed, a disease specific to that vitamin deficiency may ensue. Contrary to what my kids used to think, vitamins come from real food, not the health food store.

There is no uniform agreement among experts concerning our vitamin requirements. Differences arise because of the various methods by which requirements are determined. In addition, there is scanty data available as to how much of certain vitamins our bodies require. Recommended daily allowances (RDAs) are useful guides to quantify vitamin need, yet many experts feel these values don't accurately estimate levels for maximal benefit. However, several factors can affect how much or which type of vitamins we need at any particular time. For example, genetic variations, specific disease states, certain drugs, relative proportions of other dietary intake, food additives, environmental stresses, growth rate, and whether you have been accosted by a multilevel marketer selling Mega-Vita Super Pills all can determine your individual daily need.

"Suboptimal folic acid levels, along with suboptimal levels of vitamins B6 and B12, are a risk factor for cardiovascular disease, neural tube defects, and colon and breast cancer; low levels of vitamin D contribute to osteopenia and fractures; and low levels of the antioxidant vitamins (vitamins A, E, and C) may increase risk for several chronic diseases. Most people do not consume an optimal amount of all vitamins by diet alone. . . . It appears prudent for all adults to take vitamin supplements."

—Drs. Robert H. Fletcher and Kathleen M. Fairfield, both affiliated with Harvard Medical School

Vitamins are not only necessary for our health maintenance, but they also help prevent diseases associated with nutritional deficiencies. Vitamins give us healthy bones and teeth and prevent us from going blind and from being prone to unexpected bleeding. Vitamins also protect our hearts from damage and protect us against some forms of cancer. Recent research also suggests that high doses of vitamin C and E may reduce the risk of developing Alzheimer's disease, though more study needs to be done in this area before any recommendations can be made.

The best way to supply your body with proper vitamins is through nutritious food and not by stopping at the local health food store and spending a small fortune. If you always eat a balanced diet, you don't need any supplements. However, to counteract those times we fall short, supplements are helpful. For example, vitamin E (800 IU) has been shown in several studies to reduce menopausal hot flashes by 70 to 80 percent in some women. Furthermore, we often need much higher doses of vitamins than we can get in a balanced diet to derive maximum health benefits. For example, the doses of vitamins C and E recommended to prevent Alzheimer's disease are many times more than their respective RDAs (recommended daily allowances). Most multivitamin combinations contain only a fraction of the vitamins needed to help alleviate a particular symptom, yet they can be helpful as a supplement to an otherwise less-than-ideal diet.

As mentioned earlier, some vitamins are water soluble (the B-group and C vitamins); they are not stored in the body and are excreted in urine. We must, therefore, replenish our supplies of these vitamins daily to have sufficient amounts for our needs. Be a critical consumer. Not all vitamin supplements are useful, and you may end up lighter in the wallet and with very expensive urine!

Should you and your family take a vitamin supplement? It *is* helpful to have somewhat of a backup in today's world of nutritionally deplete processed and fast foods. So taking a single multivitamin daily can fill some gaps. However, a vitamin tablet should never be seen as a substitute for good nutrition. There are many good multivitamins available, with minimal difference in quality. The biggest difference is price, and there is little justification for this difference solely due to variations in quality. Beware of any diet or nutritional program that claims a particular vitamin or supplement is "essential." All vitamins are essential, and most of what you will see in this type of claim is marketing hype. (See chapter 9, "Beware: Snake Oil, Scams, and Rubber Wraps.")

MINERALS

Minerals are inorganic elements that are found in both living and non-living things. Once a mineral is absorbed into a plant or animal, it becomes biologically bound into the organic plant or animal system. Certain minerals are vital components of the human system, composing 4 to 5 percent of total body weight. Although only relatively small amounts of minerals are required, they are absolutely essential to normal mental and physical functioning. The body's only source for minerals is the diet. It must provide an adequate daily supply to maintain optimum health and fitness.

Minerals required in amounts greater than 100 milligrams (mg) are called macrominerals. If less than 100 mg are needed for normal functioning, they are called either microminerals or trace minerals. In some cases, we're talking only minute quantities. Macros include calcium, potassium, sodium phosphorus, magnesium, and sulfur. Micros include zinc, copper, iodine, iron, and manganese. Trace minerals include selenium, molybdenum, nickel, vanadium, chromium, cobalt, and silicon.

Did You Know?

Calcium supplementation has long been touted as a way to thwart osteoporosis in post-menopausal women. But magnesium and boron are two additional minerals that also are critical in maintaining good bone health.

Minerals trigger enzymes, like an ignition key for a car. The key may be tiny by comparison, but the car is useless without it. Minerals and enzymes work together to control the responses of our muscles, the electrical impulses that surge endlessly through our nervous systems, the beating of our hearts, the delicate balance of our body fluids, and many other complex events that must occur to maintain life.

The functions of many minerals and vitamins are interrelated. For instance, phosphorus must be present for B-complex vitamins to be absorbed; calcium could not be absorbed without vitamin D; and vitamin C enhances the absorption of iron. Minerals also provide the strength to our skeletal structure and are important factors in digestion, the formation of antibodies, and the production of hormones. Without the proper amount of minerals in the body, the vitamins we consume could not even be used at all.

Mineral deficiencies are actually more common than vitamin deficiencies. Essential vitamins are present in foods in about the same amounts around the world; however, this is not true of minerals. The mineral content of food depends on the minerals available in the soil. They could be abundant in Peoria and scarce in Pascagoula.

The human body does not efficiently break down and absorb minerals. In some foods, minerals are found in compounds that prevent absorption. Spinach, for example, is rich in calcium, but not in a form the body can utilize and is therefore just eliminated as waste.

No wonder Popeye had weak bones! Of all the minerals we consume, only a small fraction are actually absorbed. Other factors inhibiting absorption include age, gender, stress, physical activity, environment, and genetics.

Unfortunately, some of the richest sources of minerals are also loaded with calories, such as dairy products. Processed and refined foods, while loaded with calories, are virtually devoid of minerals. In addition, the United States Department of Agriculture (USDA) has been warning for decades about the consequences of mineral-depleted soils on American farms. Some of you may need a daily increase in minerals, especially pregnant women, people on certain medications, people on low-calorie diets, and vegetarians.

> **True or False?**
> Almost half of your adult bone mass was formed when you were a teenager.
> True. Healthy bones are the reason that teens need plenty of calcium! Even when teens stop growing taller, their bones continue to grow more strong and dense. Teens—especially girls—who don't consume enough calcium put their bones at risk for the rest of their lives.
> Source: *American Dietetic Association's Complete Food and Nutrition Guide*

There is reason to believe that prudent supplementation could have a positive effect on the immune system, reduce the risk of disease, and help to maintain bones, health, and fitness in general. The scientific community is feverishly investigating these possibilities.

THE BOTTOM LINE

Needless to say, this is not a complete course in the basic building blocks of nutrition, but as stated previously, understanding nutrition is critical to being able to make intelligent decisions about your health. This gives you a foundation to build on; some practical insight into viewing nutrition as a key part of a healthy lifestyle.

Bottom line: be moderate and don't obsess. Proper nutrition is a combination of knowledge, discipline, and desire—the knowledge of what is needed and how to achieve it, the discipline for persistence with restraint, and the desire to see it through. Guard against becoming the diet demon, walking around with your clipboard and calculator, figuring out the calorie content of every ounce of food. Be reasonable and acknowledge that simple rules like moderation, limiting calories, and staying balanced provide all you need to eat well. To stay healthy and lose weight, eat a balanced diet low in fat, low in sugar, and high in fiber. These are concepts you can teach your children. Show them a food label and make sure they understand what it means. That alone will put them well ahead of most of their peers.

TUBBY NATION

We are a nation of poor eaters. Go back and review the horrifying statistics from chapter one. The nutrition habits that are formed in the early years influence us throughout our lives. Many of you have a child or teenager that respects your opinion (I realize including teenagers here is stretching reality), and you can have a major impact on their eating habits. The two most powerful teaching tools at your bidding are the grocery cart and how *you* eat. In other words, your example!

Doughnuts in Dixie

Nine of the ten states with the highest rates of obesity are in the South, with Mississippi leading the way in chunkiness!

Source: *Trust for America's Health*

Good nutrition begins at the store. If you don't bring it home, you and the kids won't eat it. Take your children to the local farmer's market and show them how to pick good produce. Involve them in the selection and preparation of food. You must model good eating habits to have an impact on those around you.

Dr. Andrew Weil is a well-known advocate of family nutrition. Because of his sound nutritional advice, I quote him at various places in this book; however, I again caution you to focus on only this area of his expertise. Occasionally he strays into New Age-like philosophy in his writings, and I certainly don't imply any association with those aberrant beliefs. Dr. Weil advises, "Buying and preparing your own food also gives you the chance to influence the health of your whole family for the better. Creating family traditions of healthy eating is one of the most important things you can do for your children, whose food preferences form early in life and who will be subjected to tremendous pressure from peers and from advertising to make unhealthy choices. Involve children in food preparation whenever they show interest; talk to them about food; and help them understand that healthy eating is the cornerstone of a healthy lifestyle, that it will make them strong, energetic, and attractive. Teach them that even small changes in diets can make big differences."[13]

GETTING THE FAMILY INVOLVED

- Allow each kid to help plan his or her "night" in the weekly menu before doing the shopping. When shopping, the children can do their meal plan selection and learn label reading and price comparison. They can also be involved in the meal preparation on their night.

- Plan snacks ahead too, just like meals: veggies and dip, fresh fruit salad, cheese and crackers.

- Teach kids to choose by varying rich colors when choosing nutrient-filled fruits and veggies.

- Praise them for healthy choices and efforts made in the meal planning, and keep it fun!

- To avoid having a handy-dandy-candy battle at the checkout line during weekly shopping trips, challenge the children to pick a snack while in the produce department.

- Encourage drinking water and add a slice of fruit for flavor.

- Sometimes food can be your greatest medicine. Prevention is always better than treatment. Food can keep you healthy . . . or make you sick. I prefer to look to proper nutrition as the greatest prevention tool God has given us.

"So, what do I need to eat to be healthy?"

✗ Eat a balanced diet . . . remember the four food groups? It turns out they make sense!

✗ Eat low-fat foods . . . < 3 grams/serving.

✗ Eat low-sugar foods . . . < 6 grams/serving.

✗ Eat high-fiber foods . . . > 5 grams/serving.

✗ Adjust your total calorie consumption to your activity level, and divide your intake to about 50 percent low-glycemic carbs, 30 percent protein, and 20 percent fat.

—— FAT-PROOF POINTERS ——

Proper nutrition is the cornerstone of almost all our health issues.

In our hurry-up, fast-food, genetically altered world, healthy nutrition often continues to take a backseat.

To master a subject such as nutrition, you must understand the language.

Everything we eat for fuel can be broken down into six categories: water, carbohydrates, fats, proteins, vitamins, and minerals.

Learn to read labels correctly.

Proteins are the building blocks for muscles, tissues, and organs.

Carbohydrates are our major source of energy.

Fats, also known as lipids, act as a magnificently concentrated source of energy.

There is no uniform agreement among experts concerning our vitamin requirements.

Although only relatively small amounts of minerals are required, they are absolutely essential to normal mental and physical functioning.

Bottom line: Be moderate and don't obsess.

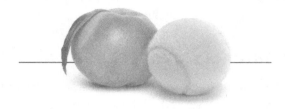

FOOD FOR THE SOUL

WHAT **THE BIBLE SAYS** ABOUT HEALTHY EATING

"Mom, do I have to go tonight? I'm really, really tired," pleaded Andy, a ten-year-old looking for a reprise from his youth group's Bible study.

"I see you weren't too tired to play Xbox," countered his mom, Marilyn.

"That's different, and you know it. It's fun and Bible study is work!"

"So you are too tired for work but not fun, right?" Marilyn said.

"Okay, busted! But I just don't feel like going tonight," whined Andy.

"Let me ask you something, Andy. How much fun would that football game on Xbox be if you didn't know the rules?"

"It would be lousy; you can't play without the rules."

Marilyn seized the teachable moment. "You know, every day is like that. If we don't know the rules, it's hard to have fun. And guess where we find out the rules?"

"The Internet, of course!" Andy teased.

"Right, you rascal. Actually, we get those rules from the Bible. It's our road map. So look at Bible study tonight as learning ways to have fun and play by the rules."

"I wonder if they make an Xbox game about Jonah and the whale," Andy said with a chuckle.

ELECTRONICALLY CHALLENGED

Yesterday I went to a local electronics store and bought a fancy new DVD recorder/player. I had been saving for this "must-have" toy for a month. I finally resolved the guilt surrounding buying it (that's a whole other discussion) and selected a model with lots of bells and whistles. For men, and some women, bragging rights no longer revolve around the size of your house or the horsepower in your car's engine, but rather the size of your hard drive or the complexity of your electronic playthings. As I gleefully opened the box and pulled out the main component, I was suddenly struck by the relative simplicity of the machine. I vividly remember my first stereo system in the early '70s. (Yes, I was a mere infant then!) Those "ancient" artifacts known as record players, which used only strange vinyl discs called records, had more wires and tubes than a telephone switchboard. You knew it was fancy because it had so many parts, and it weighed a ton.

Today, with microprocessors and integrated chips, technicians have mastered the deception of simple on the outside yet complex on the inside. After looking over my new toy, I proceeded to do what 95 percent of the population does when they get a new electronic device. I plugged it in, hit the On/Off button, and clapped joyfully as its red digital display exploded into action. Understand that at no point had I opened the owner's manual or even attempted to read any of the instructions. For I was a man, a hunter–gatherer—a conqueror—who intuitively knew that reading instructions was a sign of weakness. To my joy and amazement, the compartment that held the DVD automatically opened and I gingerly placed my *Passion of the Christ* DVD in the slot. (In some warped rationalization, I thought I could justify the purchase of this machine by starting with a religious video.) The cartridge retracted into the component like a turtle pulling its head into its shell and then . . . nothing. Not even the opening credits appeared on the screen. Fighting the urge to throw the DVD player out the window, I finally did what I should have done even before the Styrofoam packing was tossed aside.

I read the owner's manual.

Painfully I trudged from page one all the way to page thirty-six. It was all that I could endure and still be true to my manliness. Yet I was amazed. I was absolutely spellbound by the unbelievable things this DVD player could do. Without the owner's manual, I would be relegated to a machine that permanently functioned at a baseline level. No doubt I would have been haunted by the annoying 12:00 image forever blinking and mocking me whenever I glanced in its direction. Now, with the owner's manual in hand, I could play surround sound, record, bookmark, skip, reverse, fast-forward, and even put subtitles in Mandarin Chinese. A whole new world of electronic bliss was suddenly opened up, revealing fascinating options and possibilities. How? Simply by reading the guidebook. The owner's manual took me from being a mechanical moron to becoming an electronic wizard with minimal pain and effort.

OWNER'S MANUAL

The Bible is our owner's manual for life. God didn't just deposit us on earth to flounder around, aimlessly trudging through an evolutionary maze to randomly find our way. He gave us very specific instructions as to how to live, love, eat, exercise, remain healthy, and cultivate a relationship with him. But just like that DVD owner's manual, we have to read, absorb, and apply the Bible for it to become meaningful on a personal level.

Why do we only refer to the owner's manual when we get into a mess and can't fix things? When the DVD malfunctions, then we grudgingly turn to the troubleshooting section. Likewise, so many of us resort to reading the Bible only when faced with troubles or confusion. Why is it that we turn to God's guidebook only to solve problems instead of preventing them? Doesn't it make more sense to learn to do things correctly the first time? W. Edwards Deming, the great American efficiency expert, taught Japanese and American businesspeople that it was far better to prevent defective widgets than replace them after they were already made. This simple concept revolutionized the post-war Japanese economy. This principle of excellence applies to our lives also.

Did You Know?

- ✗ Forty-nine different foods are mentioned in the Bible.

- ✗ Almonds and pistachios are the only nuts mentioned in the Bible.

- ✗ Salt is mentioned more than thirty times.

Yes, the Scriptures have a troubleshooting function. They provide much comfort and counsel in times of crisis, but if we focus on corrective remedies alone, we will miss an incredible opportunity to learn how to live joyfully and abundantly on a daily basis.

Soon you will discover that no fad diet, miracle drug, exercise machine, or surgical procedure can be as comprehensive a solution to fat-proofing your family as God's Owner's Manual. The wisdom in its pages proves to be as timeless and as applicable to health and wellness today as it was in centuries past. Bible study is one cog in the wheel of the healing triad of mind, body, and spirit. It addresses specific spiritual needs that are frequently ignored in the healing process.

STORMS OF LIFE

Scripture is so much more than just do's and don'ts. It is the foundation upon which our lives are built. I heard the following story—I'm not sure of the author—that illustrates the importance of Scripture. Years ago, a farmer owned land along the Atlantic seacoast. He constantly advertised for hired hands since most people were reluctant to work on area farms because they dreaded the awful storms that raged across the ocean, wreaking havoc on buildings and crops. The farmer interviewed numerous applicants but received a steady stream of refusals. Finally, a short, thin man, well past middle age, approached the farmer. "Are you a good farmhand?" the farmer asked him. "Well, I can sleep when the wind blows," answered the little man. Although puzzled by this answer, the farmer, desperate for help, hired him. The little man worked well around the farm, busy from dawn to dusk, and the farmer felt satisfied with the man's work.

Then one night the wind howled loudly in from offshore. Jumping out of bed, the farmer grabbed a lantern and rushed next door to the hired hand's sleeping quarters. He shook the little man and yelled, "Get up! A storm is coming! Tie things down before they blow away!" The little man rolled over in bed and said firmly, "No, sir. I told you, I can sleep when the wind blows." Enraged by the response, the farmer was tempted to fire him on the spot. Instead, he hurried outside to prepare for the storm. To his amazement, he discovered that all of the haystacks had been covered with tarpaulins. The cows were in the barn, the chickens were in the coops, and the doors were barred. The shutters were tightly secured. Everything was tied down so nothing would blow away. The farmer then understood what his hired hand meant, so he himself returned to his bed to also sleep while the wind blew.

When you're prepared—spiritually, mentally, and physically—you have nothing to fear. We secure ourselves against the storms of life by grounding ourselves in the Word of God. The storms will come and strong winds will blow across our lives—be it sickness, stress, or emotional turmoil—so shelter your family by having a firm understanding of God's Word.

A GOD WHO HEALS

In the beginning, God established his predilection for health, wellness, and healing. In Exodus 15:26, he says, "If you will listen carefully to the voice of the Lord your God and do what is right in his sight, obeying his commands and laws, then I will not make you suffer the diseases I sent on the Egyptians; for I am the Lord who heals you."

Here God calls himself *Yahweh Rapha*—the God who heals. This passage is especially significant because it comes in response to the grumbling of the Israelites against Moses. They had been traveling in the desert for three days without water and finally arrived at an area know as Mara, and there they found water; however, it was brackish, tainted, and undrinkable. The people were distraught and complained bitterly. In response to Moses' pleading, God miraculously transformed the water into sweet and nourishing refreshment. Then God issued a challenge. If the Israelites will listen to his admonitions and do as he instructs, they will not suffer any of the diseases of the Egyptians. These instructions are like a lamppost illuminating *our* path toward better health.

You may be wondering, *Big deal, I haven't been overly concerned about any Egyptian diseases lately.* However, if you look at the historical context of the times, the relevance to our own times becomes more apparent. Originally, the Egyptians were a predominately agrarian society, but as they began to prosper and rule other lands, they became avid consumers of many delicacies and extravagant dishes. This included primarily meat, which had been in somewhat short supply. It was also known that the Egyptians perfected the skills of fermentation and produced a variety of alcohol-laden products. With this radical shift in dietary habits, the wealthy Egyptians began to experience a weakening change in their physical well-being. This fact is well documented in both ancient writings and in the well preserved, mummified remains of Egyptian nobility. In fact, evidence of atherosclerosis, stiffness of the joints, dental decay, and premature death have all been confirmed by autopsies of ancient bodies. God was not only challenging and admonishing the Israelites, but also giving them practical advice on proper nutritional intake. This advice is wise to heed in today's society, where one out of every two adults will die of heart disease!

This verse in Exodus also gives clear instructions for following God's will in many diverse situations. **Step one** is to *listen carefully—* pay attention and avail yourself of what is written and spoken by God through the Holy Spirit. Whether it is healthy nutrition, exercise, surgery, medicines, or vitamins, God is the source of all. But if you are unable or unwilling to listen, this advice and instruction will fall on deaf ears. God granted us two ears and one mouth so we would listen twice as much as we speak. If we heed what God tells us in Scripture, then we will indeed be blessed. **Step two** is to *act obediently* on what we read and hear.

KNOWING IS GOOD, DOING IS BETTER

Knowledge is only part of the equation in understanding the relevance of what the Bible says about nutrition. It is one thing to hear or see the instructions; it's quite another to carry them out. God places a premium on not just hearing the word, but doing what it says. We have a responsibility to do both what is good for our family's health and to avoid what is harmful.

Does this mean God's blessings are conditional, depending solely on our actions? Absolutely not! God's love for us and his desire for us to be healthy is not the result of some spiritual lottery of chance, and it's not doled out to only those who earn it. It is available to all. But since we have free will, we can choose to pursue healthy practices or choose to embrace unhealthy lifestyles. God is plainly stating that if we will hear and understand his instructions and then apply them daily, our lives will be less plagued with disease and tribulation. He doesn't say we will never be sick; that would contradict his natural law. It also doesn't imply that we are solely responsible for bringing on cancers, for example, by our own actions. That instills unhealthy guilt and is misplaced. It does mean that we play an important role in our family's health. Neither are we totally subject to the random whims of nature. Even the child who is born with a congenital heart problem—surely not the result of his unhealthy lifestyle choices—can benefit by adopting some of the healthy recommendations from Scripture.

> Throughout history the spiritual leader in a community was also often the "healer" or physician. It is only in the last three hundred years that the purviews of spirituality and health have been separated.

Even the righteous, the pious, and the faithful get sick. We all know those people who exercise regularly, eat a healthy diet, and are never stressed, yet they still develop heart disease! Family genes, the effects of cultural mores, and the impact of the environment must also be considered. One of my favorite bumper stickers states, "Eat healthy. Exercise daily. Die anyway!" Cynical but true. Nevertheless, I might add that those families who eat well and exercise daily will, on average, die later than those who don't, and will have a better quality of life while living!

Even those who appear healthiest get sick from time to time. We don't instantly become immune from all illness and disease by following a magical set of ordained guidelines. The reality is that all of us—young, old, Christian, Hindu, male, female, rich, poor, real blondes, fake blondes—are subject to accidents, viruses, microbes, and other nasty little things. That is the world in which God places us.

PART OF THE SOLUTION

The Bible is very specific in teaching that good nutrition is critical in maintaining health. Physical nourishment is important, but not in isolation. I have said that food plays a role in the overall fitness equation, but it is only a part of the solution.

Most of what you need to know for healthy living—from nutrition, to stress management, to spiritual salvation—is contained in the Scriptures. Although the Bible doesn't give . . .

. . . a dosage for antibiotics;

. . . a design for a CT scan machine;

. . . or a specific recipe for tofu ravioli;

. . . it does admonish you to seek out wise counsel when you are sick. It does show God working in the lives of his people. It does teach you to rely on the advice of learned friends (such as your physician), and it does tell you to study what God's Word has to say about nutrition and emotional wellness.

OLD TESTAMENT ADVICE

Leviticus 11 contains many of the Jewish laws of food purity. Many of these proclamations were designed both to provide a separate identity for the Jews and to keep them healthy by forbidding the consumption of certain foods. For example, animals that were noted to be scavengers were labeled as unclean and not fit to eat. This had a practical application as it protected the people from a common means of disease transmission. The pig, a notorious scavenger, eats whatever it can find, including dead animals and garbage, so avoiding pork was a means of avoiding such harmful diseases as trichinosis and other bacterial infestations.

NEW TESTAMENT EYES

Jesus, on the other hand, brings a different perspective to many of the Old Testament laws. He knew that the Pharisees mistakenly trusted only in the laws to declare man's fitness before God. The Pharisees taught that a man could be clean and holy by simply keeping the Law of Moses and its corollaries and avoiding certain foods. Jesus saw this false piety as a barrier for people to understand the grace of God. He taught that following such dietary prescriptions may keep you free from some health problems and show your outward obedience to God, yet it could not grant you salvation. Jesus taught that it is not what we put into our mouth that affects our character, but it is what comes out of our mouth that signifies who we are. Our character is an inside job. Jesus knew that what makes a person unclean are evil thoughts, malice, deceit, lewdness, arrogance, and folly—not a big slab of bacon. Always go back to wholeness: the concept of health as a balance of mind, body, and spirit. Lard may be bad for the heart, but not as bad as an unforgiving spirit!

A HOLY SMORGASBORD

Just as God created man and woman for each other, so he created certain foodstuffs to be consumed. Look at Genesis 1:29–30: "And God said, 'Look! I have given you the seed-bearing plants throughout the earth and all the fruit trees for your food. And I have given all the grasses and other green plants to the animals and birds for their food.'"

This is not too tough to figure out! God says that a predominately vegetarian diet is healthy and it is what he designed for us to use as fuel. Anyone who is familiar with current nutritional research can tell you a diet based on fruits, vegetables, and plants is one of the healthiest around. Dr. Dean Ornish has become well-known for his studies showing how a vegetarian diet can prevent heart disease.

He has taken this a step further and has shown convincingly that the proper diet can actually reverse preexisting heart disease.

The verses in Genesis establish "seed-bearing plants" as healthy food. This includes grains, beans, legumes, nuts, seeds, vegetables, fruits, herbs, and spices. The variety of good foods is vast. Dr. Colin Campbell says, "The evidence now amassed from researchers around the world shows that a plant-based diet is good for the prevention of cancer and for the prevention of heart disease, as well as obesity, diabetes, cataracts, macular degeneration, Alzheimer's, cognitive dysfunction, multiple sclerosis, osteoporosis, and other diseases."[1]

Did You Know?

Not only is there too much fat in meat, it's the wrong kind. Nearly half the fat in meat is the artery-clogging, saturated type. And, of course, meat is also high in cholesterol. Beef fat is more saturated than poultry fat because the bacteria in the ruminant stomach of cattle hydrogenate, or saturate, the fats in the plants that cows eat. It's like having a fat factory inside the food source!

In twenty years of researching and reading about nutrition, I have never seen a single study that negated the beneficial effects of a vegetarian-based diet. In fact, we are in the midst of an explosion of scientific literature supporting what the Bible recommended centuries ago. Jesus and his disciples were not vegetarians. They ate fish and other meats, but they exhibited balance in their food choices. Critics say Jesus was only following the regional traditional dietary habits and that scholars are reading too much into the daily details of their lives. I disagree. I feel it is just exactly what Jesus and the disciples did on a regular basis that forms a guide for our behavior. It is not productive to play the "what if" game. *"What if Jesus had lived in a different geographic area and eaten only cheese and sausage, would that be all you say to eat now?"* The point is that Jesus lived where he did and lived at the time he did for reasons known only to God. But the historical fact remains that he was a first-century Jew in Judea, and I believe it was no accident. What Jesus and the disciples did has significance whether it was a daily ritual or a miraculous healing. That is one of the miracles of Scripture—its transcendence and application across time and cultures.

BALANCE

Nevertheless, it is important to keep in perspective the guidelines from the Jewish dietary laws. Remember, God is stating that these foods are good. That doesn't imply that others are necessarily bad. We, as Christians, must view this information through the lens of New Testament teachings. Those who proclaim that Scripture teaches we should all be strict vegetarians haven't read all of Scripture. One great pitfall of biblical interpretation is to selectively choose passages that support a particular point of view, while ignoring other teachings that appear to give a different perspective. This is illustrated by those who use only the Pentateuch, and more specifically Leviticus, as their basis for dietary guidance.

Healthy Foods of the Bible

Here are some common foods that are specifically mentioned as healthy in the Old Testament.

Honey	Nuts
Fowl	Figs
Beans	Herbs
Grapes	Bread
Fish	Cucumbers
Melons	Lentils
Raisins	Fruit
Barley	Spices
Vegetables	Cheese
Olives	Grain
Vinegar	Garlic

Adapted from *What the Bible Says About Healthy Living,* Russell, 1996

Note: This is not a comprehensive list; I limited it to items that we commonly consume in the United States. And remember, everything in moderation, nothing in excess . . . even the good stuff!

The whole of Scripture is clear on nutrition: amounts matter (gluttony is a sin), variety is good (God's abundance), and balance is necessary (mind, body, and spirit).

CLEAN AND UNCLEAN

Besides eating a plant-based diet, the Bible also addresses the eating of meat. God in his wisdom gave instructions to Noah about how to live differently after the flood. "All the wild animals, large and small, and all the birds and fish will be afraid of you. I have placed them in your power. I have given them to you for food, just as I have given you grain and vegetables. But you must never eat animals that still have their lifeblood in them" (Genesis 9:2–4).

God gives more specific instructions in Deuteronomy 14:4–20, as he explained the laws for designating animals as "clean" or "unclean." God states it is permissible to eat "clean" animals and forbidden to consume the "unclean." Why the difference?

In today's language it would be a simplistic assumption to believe that God was commanding man to stay away from dirty food. That may be true, but that is not the correct interpretation of these biblical terms. According to scholars, a clean animal is defined by what it eats and the cleanliness of its digestive tract. If you refer to the laws in Deuteronomy, the only clean animals are those that have divided hooves and chew their cud. It is no surprise that the only animals that fit both categories are those that consume mainly plants. The scavengers and the flesh eaters are considered unclean. The group of unclean animals is called omnivores, because they literally will eat anything. What an animal consumed, in turn, would be reflected in what a person ate. This prohibition from consuming unclean animals protected the Israelites from many of the diseases that were transmitted by means of bacteria and parasites. Examples of clean animals are calves, deer, goat, ox, sheep, and duck. Examples of unclean animals are crab, catfish, shrimp, pigs, rabbit, ostrich, squirrel, oyster, and lobster.

Does this distinction apply in today's world of strict manufacturing standards and quality control? Absolutely! The benefit in excluding the "unclean" animals today is not derived from the standpoint of communicable diseases, but from the avoidance of the consequences of high saturated fat diets. A list of unclean animals is populated by those whose meat is among the highest in saturated fats, a known risk factor for heart disease.

Another rationale for the clean and unclean designation had little to do with nutrition. As has been discussed, many of the dietary laws of Moses were designed to provide the Israelites with a separate identity. It made them different from their neighbors and preserved the integrity of their culture. Their eating habits distinguished them from other people. It was also a part of developing the discipline to obey God and his commands.

Does the distinction between clean and unclean relate in any way to your spiritual maturity? Are you a better Christian if you limit your food intake to clean animals versus unclean ones? Let me say that abiding by these dietary laws does not imply any greater degree of spiritual attainment, piety, or salvation. You don't achieve spiritual cleanliness by keeping certain dietary laws. One of the principal problems Jesus had with the Pharisees was their obsession with strict adherence to dietary laws. The law actually became a stumbling block on their path to righteousness. The Pharisees worshiped the law instead of the law Giver. Following these dietary guidelines is a discipline, not a ticket to heaven.

In his letters, the apostle Paul says eating clean or unclean animals does not have any spiritual value itself; however, the reason to follow these instructions is to glorify God by being obedient and acknowledging his desire and design for our health.

GLUTTONY

A tremendous variety of foods are available that are specifically blessed by God. These foods are abundant, and when used properly, will provide the cornerstone of any healthy lifestyle. However, you must be ever vigilant about excesses. You can get fat by eating only the "right" foods. Too much of the good stuff can be bad for you, your family, and your waistline. Forgive the repetition, but amounts count!

Dr. S. I. McMillen writes in his bestseller *None of These Diseases:*

The Bible has many warnings against intemperate eating habits. Many times gluttons and drunkards are mentioned in the same verse. One such verse says: "Do not join those who drink too much wine or gorge themselves on meat" (Proverbs 23:20). Christians have been among the first to condemn alcoholic beverages, but I have seldom heard sermons addressed to the sin of gluttony. Although this sin is common among members of almost every church in the land, most preachers— especially those who wish to keep their positions beyond the current year—continue to ignore the biblical injunctions against overeating. For millions of Christians, however, obedience to these biblical warnings would fortify character, improve appearance, revive happiness, renew efficiency, restore health, and increase longevity.[2]

MEALS MATTER

The experience of the earliest Christians was often punctuated by meals. For them, meals represented intimacy and joy of family, fellowship, and friends. Meal gatherings for believers became places where the power and presence of Christ was manifest. The best example is in the observance of the Last Supper. Here the mystery of the suffering and resurrection of Jesus was represented by bread and wine. The bread and the cup provide the tools for the remembrance of the ultimate sacrifice. Truly, there can be no greater example of the celebration of a meal. Indeed, it was a meal celebrating the meal of the Old Testament Exodus (Passover). Whenever we celebrate communion, we come to God's table and humbly recall what grace really means.

> "People tend to think of breakthroughs in medicine as a new drug, a laser, or a high-tech surgical procedure. They often have a hard time believing that the simple choices that we make in our lifestyle—what we eat, how we respond to stress, whether or not we smoke cigarettes, how much exercise we get, and the quality of our relationships and support—can be as powerful as drugs and surgery. But they often are."
>
> —Dr. Dean Ornish,
> *Stress, Diet, and Your Heart*

Jesus spoke often of being the bread of life, and wine was used extensively in analogies and teachings. The sacredness of the table was punctuated by using meals as times of both worship and remembrance. Paul addresses the importance of the shared meal in his letter to the Corinthians: "What I meant was that you are not to associate with anyone who claims to be a Christian yet indulges in sexual sin, or is greedy, or worships idols, or is abusive, or a drunkard, or a swindler. Don't even eat with such people" (1 Corinthians 5:11). In ancient times, who you ate with was often more important than who you slept with, according to New Testament scholar Luke Timothy Johnson. He states that it is significant that one of the few times Paul actually quotes Jesus in his letters is in regard to a meal, the Last Supper.[3] Meals and the gatherings associated with meals played a significant role in the development of early Christianity, and today meals continue to be an integral part of church fellowship.

THEOLOGY OF FOOD

The theology of food—the study of how food is used in the context of Scripture—is fascinating. Both Old and New Testaments are filled with references to food, and there is a great deal we can learn from both texts. Just as other stories, parables, and teachings are applicable to us today, so the importance and symbolism of food in Scripture can mirror uses in the family's life.

In the Old Testament, food is used largely in terms of worship and fellowship. Some rituals of worship included altars, which began as sacrificial tables. Abraham began the tradition by building several altars at which he served up sacrifices to God as one of the first symbols of worship. One of the earliest stories in Genesis describes the different sacrifices of Cain and Abel, both using common sources of food. So from the outset, we see the importance of food as a symbol and tool of worship.

Part of that worship is the understanding of our dependence on God for our continued existence. Without food, we will not survive, and God is the source and provider of that sustenance. As a form of worship, we offer back to God that which he has given to us. This acknowledges our trust in God for our most basic needs. Communion of the bread and wine—the gifts of God for the people of God— is maintained through food shared before him and food shared with his people. Food is celebrated when it is used in worship. This is especially pertinent today when we celebrate God's grace and our abundance.

Leviticus gives special instructions for feasts that were meant to celebrate God through the festivals of food. These were special, regular, and corporate occasions for remembering what God had done, giving thanks to him, and rededicating lives to his service. The three main festivals in Jewish tradition—the Passover, the feast of Pentecost, and the feast of Tabernacles—were structured to gather family and friends and be in the presence of God. Even today the family dinner table should be a place for celebration, instruction, and fellowship. We don't have formal feasts, but we do have holidays that are inevitably surrounded by food. Use food as a means of thanksgiving, a tool for praise, and a way of remembrance.

The New Testament writers also embraced meals as times of special significance. The physician and author Luke highlights how meals served many roles. Levi, the tax collector, was the first to hold a dinner in honor of Jesus with the expressed purpose of evangelism. He gathered all his fellow tax collectors for a party at which Jesus was the guest of honor, and proceeded to let the occasion flow into a means for Jesus to minister to these folks. This was a despised group of "sinners" (outcasts) who may have never had any other opportunity to hear about or enter the kingdom of God. This type of forum—sharing a meal together—sets the tone for many outreach ministries today that encourage home-based dinner meetings where the Gospel is shared. Serving food to those in need also becomes an evangelism of action.

Scripture as well describes how meals could be times of confrontation. We are all familiar with the story in Luke 7 where Jesus is at a meal with some Pharisees and a woman of questionable character anoints his feet with oil. It is hard to imagine today what an incredible scene this was at the time, but picture a formal banquet at your local convention center ballroom. The room is filled with local politicians and dignitaries from the business and religious community. A professor of rabbinical studies and other honored guests are sitting at the head table, and all of a sudden, through the crowd walks a known prostitute. She runs up to the Rabbi and gingerly pours olive oil on his patent leather shoes. Now, I would dare say that the majority of the attendees would be aghast, and I suspect the emcee would already be on the phone to security. But suddenly and quite unexpectedly, the Rabbi gently places his hand on the girl's head and tells her she is a woman of enormous kindness and thanks her for her act of humility. I can only speculate as to the conversation surrounding the rest of the meal. Likewise, Jesus did the unexpected. He often used meals and gatherings as times of confrontation and teaching.

The feeding of the five thousand is another occasion where food played an important symbolic role in teaching. Jesus met not only an immediate physical need but also used the opportunity to talk of spiritual food. This was a training ground for the disciples as they saw in words and deeds the very embodiment of the love of God.

One of Jesus' greatest teachings about discipleship is found in Luke 14. As was the custom, a person's place at the banquet table signified their rank or position of authority. The closer to the head of the table, the more important you were. Jesus used this tradition to illustrate how discipleship worked in the kingdom of God. He taught that one should never boast or seek glory, but humble yourself before God. He concludes, "For the proud will be humbled, but the humble will be honored" (verse 11).

Luke describes a scene where food plays a significant role in recognizing Jesus. After Jesus' resurrection, he encountered two travelers on the road to Emmaus. They didn't know who he was

> "It was a common saying among the Puritans, 'Brown bread and the Gospel is good fare.'"
> —Matthew Henry (1622–1714)

until "he took a small loaf of bread, asked God's blessing on it, broke it, then gave it to them. Suddenly, their eyes were opened, and they recognized him" (24:30–31). The act of giving thanks, blessing, and feeding was intimately associated with Jesus, so much so it was this act that opened the traveler's eyes to his identity.

MEALS STILL MATTER

These principles, so much a part of early Christianity and Judaism, still have clarity and relevance today. I recently watched the Steven Spielberg movie *Munich,* which details the Israeli secret service response to the terrorist massacre of athletes at the 1972 Olympics. In the final climactic scene, the leader of the Mossad retaliation team, who had been alienated from his own people, asks about reconciliation. He is speaking to his contact in the Mossad, a fellow Jew, and his way of saying "let's put our past behind us and move on" was to ask his countryman, "Can we break bread together?" The act of breaking bread together would become, for them, a powerful symbol of reconciliation. This signified the importance of sharing one's table with another. It was a moment filled with centuries of tradition, and the meaning of that simple gesture was immediately known to both men.

A meal—a table of fellowship—was and is a place of reconciliation. The family mealtime can be a sacred time, a place set apart for fellowship. Just reflecting on this image can transform how you approach each meal and would set a life-changing precedent for your children to follow.

Food is a gift from God. If we heed his admonitions, we will find health and happiness. Many principles from Scripture are wonderful in their simplicity. In Scripture, virtually every mention of food is celebrated, meals are meaningful, and moderation is rewarded. If you accept and adopt these simple precepts, you can take a major step forward in fat-proofing your family.

—— FAT-PROOF POINTERS ——

The Bible is our owner's manual for life.

We have God's own revelation as to how to live healthy, meaningful lives.

We worship a healing God.

Listen carefully, pay attention, and avail yourself of what is written and spoken by God through the Holy Spirit.

Even the righteous, the pious, and the faithful get sick.

Jesus brings a different perspective to many of the Old Testament laws.

God says that a predominately vegetarian diet is healthy and is what he designed for us to use as fuel.

Those who proclaim that Scripture teaches that we should all be strict vegetarians haven't read all of Scripture.

The whole of Scripture is clear on nutrition: gluttony is a sin, variety is good, and balance is necessary.

You don't achieve spiritual cleanliness by keeping certain dietary laws.

You *can* get fat by eating only the "right" foods.

Meal gatherings for believers became places where the power and presence of Christ was manifest.

In the Old Testament, food is used largely in terms of worship and fellowship.

New Testament writers also embraced meals as times of special significance.

Food is a gift from God.

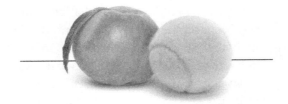

CHILDREN AND TEENS

NUTRITIONAL **SPECIFICS**

Children are not just little adults. Teens and "tweens" (generally ages ten to twelve), in particular, are a breed all to themselves. All the rules of good nutrition apply to children and adolescents, but with certain modifications. The adolescent and teen years are absolutely critical in the overall plan to fat-proof your family. Here the foundation is laid, and the habits established during the early years transfer to adulthood. We have already seen that overweight kids tend to become overweight adults, saddled with all the problems that accompany being overfat. The positive side of the equation is that kids who learn healthy fitness habits early tend to keep them imprinted on their brain for life.

It is essential to understand that you, the parent, are the single most influential person in establishing the healthy habits of your child. Modeling is a powerful teacher, and you can't expect your child to adopt a fitness-first lifestyle without your own commitment. I've said it before, but the most valuable tool you possess for teaching your kids about a healthy lifestyle is your uncommon sense.

This book is about taking common knowledge and applying it uncommonly, that is, consistently and persistently.

No doubt, the greatest challenge is to not go with the flow and allow your child to succumb to the status quo. For kids, fitting in is often a huge priority, and in today's world that often means fast food and fickle fitness. Teenagers especially have a need to blend in, and any intrusion into that space will be resisted. To most teenagers, being seen as different is about as desirable as warts; however, there are techniques you can apply to minimize the appearance of non-conformity with their peers. It's what I call disguised conformity.

Don't use the term *diet* with children or adolescents; to them that will imply restriction and generally elicit rebellion. You are teaching lifestyle changes that become permanent habits, not a yo-yo program that creates more problems than it solves. Teach them that thin doesn't necessarily translate as fit. Indeed, misunderstanding this can be the origin of some eating disorders and abnormal body image problems.

Don't overdo it! A recently published study found that frequent dieting by mothers was associated with frequent dieting by their adolescent daughters. They also found that girls with moms who had weight concerns were more likely to develop concerns about their own bodies.

Source: *Journal of the American Dietetic Association,* August 2006

This is an opportune time to reinforce the difference between fat and fit. Tweens are especially sensitive to body changes, and relegating them to diets does more harm than good. In many ways, it is a game of semantics because the term *diet* carries so much emotional baggage. For many kids, telling them to go on a diet is a direct affront to their self image, and they are not mature enough to understand the consequences. If your child is overweight—or you want to help them not become so—and you want to encourage weight loss, don't refer to your new eating program as a diet; label it as healthy eating or balanced eating. That simple shift in terminology eases the emotional impact and makes the transition more palatable. Your goal is not to have a runway-model slim family; it is to have a fit family, and hopefully you can see the difference by now.

With your children, as with you, amounts matter, variety is key, exercise is mandatory, and modeling is the best teacher. It is funda-mental to avoid severely restrictive dietary guidelines with your kids. That is a setup for failure. You must educate them on what is bad and teach them in a way (as we will explore) that facilitates their understanding and eventually leads to their own healthy choices. But more important, you must show them the abundance of good things God has provided for food and snacks.

You have to constantly navi-gate a minefield of misinforma-tion, biased reports, extreme and contradictory opinions, and con-flicting data when it comes to proper nutrition for your chil-dren. A healthy dose of reality often makes sorting out these points of view easier. Observe how your child acts and feels. Even if a particular eating approach looks healthy on the surface, if it makes your child feel poorly, there is a problem. Every child, even within the same family, is a unique indi-vidual, and his or her needs, wants, and reaction to foods can vary. Don't forget to embrace each child's individuality, and tailor an approach to his or her needs. (The next chapter contains specific guidelines—for your child and you—about eating right and losing weight.)

> **Did You Know?**
>
> Children who are overweight at age two face a five-times-higher risk of being overweight at age twelve.
>
> Source: *Pediatrics,* September 2006

HOW MUCH SHOULD YOUNGER CHILDREN EAT?

As stated before, there are some generalities that apply to virtu-ally all children and adolescents. One of the biggest problems with kids and food is portions. They just plain eat too much, and too much of the bad stuff. As with adults, amounts (calories) matter. On the opposite end of the spectrum are the kids who are picky eaters. They don't eat that much, but what they do eat is not exactly nutri-tional. This is especially a problem with younger children.

Let's consider the overeater first.

Children's stomachs are smaller, so it is logical that they need less to fill them up; yet we persist in giving adult portions to children. The constant berating to clean your plate stems from an era where food was less abundant and there was a longer time between meals. There wasn't the deluge of snack foods and fast-food establishments we have today. It makes more sense to feed children somewhat similarly to the model used by folks with diabetes. Have six small meals throughout the day as opposed to three gigantic feasts. Smaller portions of the right kind of foods keep the blood sugar levels steady and give a feeling of satiety. Realistically, many adults could benefit from this schedule also. If you keep a log of total calories consumed, you will often see that the number is less with the small, frequent meals than the traditional three-meal scenario. (See page 145 for more details about eating smaller, more frequent meals each day.)

Using Finesse With Finicky Eaters

⚡ Change Focus: Don't force a child to eat certain food; focus on table manners instead.

⚡ Divide and Conquer: Parents are responsible for what, when, and where to eat; kids control what and how much.

⚡ Plan Snacks: Eliminate grazing between meals.

⚡ Offer a Variety: Tofu will not make a child ask for seconds.

⚡ Don't Bribe: Using food as a reward often leads to poor eating habits.

Adapted from *Secrets of Feeding a Healthy Family*, by Ellyn Satter

---

PICKY EATERS

What about the finicky eater? How do you deal with the child who fixates on one type of food? My daughter, when she was about four, would have eaten macaroni and cheese for breakfast, lunch, and dinner if we had let her. (To our everlasting shame, we did in many cases.) When faced with this dilemma, keep in mind that you want to pour a foundation for a fit lifestyle based on good nutrition. Don't lose the war because you choose to fight every battle with gusto. Along those lines, never make the dinner table a combat zone. Constant bickering at the dinner table is more harmful than a plate of sugar cookies!

Parents are responsible for what food is in the house and how that food is prepared, but ultimately children control how much of it they eat. That is why education with a healthy dose of psychology is a valuable tool in your armamentarium for fat-proofing your kids. Later in this chapter, I will outline effective ways to teach kids based on their learning styles. For example, give your picky eater defined choices. Don't ask her what she wants for lunch; instead say, "Would you like a tuna sandwich or a turkey burger for lunch?" This gives her a choice but only within the parameters you set. It may be helpful to have the child participate in the preparation of the food. Not only is this a great opportunity to teach, but it gives her some ownership and a sense of independence that she craves. The pickiness in her eating may simply be a symptom of her desire for control, and that is usually not a long-term dilemma. Most kids will lose this predilection if it is not made into a huge confrontation.

In rare instances, a child's stingy eating habits may be due to an intuitive desire to avoid certain foods he or she is allergic or sensitive to. Milk allergies—where dairy products create a great deal of gastrointestinal discomfort—are on the rise. If your child exhibits a lack of interest in dairy products, it may be an early sign of such an allergy.

> **What Do Growing Teens Need?**
>
> Once a child hits puberty, both boys and girls not only become brain damaged (relax, it's a joke), but they also require more calories to fuel their explosive growth. In many instances, these children quickly become taller and larger than their parents. Even though their minds may not be at the same development level, they can now adopt many of the nutritional recommendations for adults.

A "STYLE" FOR EVERY CHILD AND TEEN

At the end of the day, fat-proofing your family is about teaching and learning. Generally, it begins with your learning with gusto about healthy nutrition and exercise, and then relaying with enthusiasm this information to your children. Occasionally, the teaching flows the other way, with kids whipping their rotund relatives into shape. We all know from past experience that teaching children and teens anything can be challenging. Communication is not a one-way street. We have to be aware of our teaching/communication styles and also the learning styles of our children. I have often found myself wondering why my thirteen-year-old doesn't grasp a concept or appreciate information like I do. And I have come to find out she feels the same bewilderment about me!

If you are to indeed take the lead in promoting fitness over fatness, you must adapt your teaching to the *learning style* of your child. If I ambled into a U.S. classroom of seventeen-year-olds and began teaching them science in Chinese, my guess is that they would not ace the SAT in that area. I could exert a Herculean effort in teaching, but it would fail miserably. So it is in attempting to teach kids about health and fitness. You have to speak a language that they understand and teach in a manner that allows them to use their God-given abilities to comprehend.

Some children are visual learners; show them pictures of good foods, or the foods themselves. Take them to sporting events where they can see athletes in action. Actively involve them in preparing meals. Some children respond more to verbal teachings. Spend time telling them stories of everyday people who have lost weight, or talk about ways to increase fitness. Take time to listen to your child. Often children will provide clues to their learning style by the manner of their speech. Visual kids will say things like, "I see what you mean," "I see that clearly," or "I can see your point." Verbal kids say things like, "I hear where you are coming from" or "That sounds good to me." Most kids (and adults) are able to cross over and utilize both types of learning, but generally one dominates. Determining how your child and spouse process information can make teaching about health and fitness—or anything—that much more effective.

Now, let's take an average day and break it down into its nutritional components for children and teens. Use this information to coax your kids into wellness. Before they actually know they are doing something healthy, it's too late—the habits are being reinforced. It is stealth learning!

BREAK THE FAST

Breakfast, or break the fast, is the cornerstone in building a healthy nutritional lifestyle for your child. The typical family will have ten to eleven hours between dinner and breakfast, so skipping this essential meal will add an additional three to five hours to this fast. This duration of fasting forces the body to shoot fatty acids into the bloodstream, as part of the natural fasting metabolism. These are the same fatty acids that are responsible for atherosclerotic changes (hardening of the arteries) in blood vessels. You may be thinking, *So what. Heart disease is a problem in adults, not kids.* Wrong! Medical studies, some done on children as young as fourteen, are finding that heart damage may actually begin early in life. Just like adults, it is critical that your child have a nutritional breakfast to fuel up for the day and to set the metabolic tone for the next twenty-four hours. Breakfast is not to be skipped, nor is it meant to create blood sugar levels that make syrup jealous.

The chief barrier to healthy breakfasts in my house is time. It seems as if every morning, especially during the school year, is a race against the clock. "Where's my homework?" "Is my jean skirt dry?" "I can't find the curling iron!" (Can you tell I live in a household flooded with estrogen?) To buy time in the morning, I naively began setting the alarm a few minutes earlier. That worked for about two days, and then it was back to the herding-cats scenario. The most practical solutions we have discovered are quick, healthy choices. For example, a piece of fruit and a cup of low-fat yogurt is relatively quick to eat and begins the day with a great energy source. Another good idea is to whip up a fruit smoothie the day before and let it chill overnight for quick consumption the next morning. Even some (I emphasize *some*) cereals can be quick and healthy.

ARE YOUR KIDS SWEET ON CEREAL?

Now, let's look at a few guidelines for buying cereals, the staple in many household breakfast agendas. In general, if it contains a toy, comic book, spy ring, or anything plastic, odds are the cereal can't stand on its own merits. You wouldn't buy a steak just because it had a free lipstick case stuck through its middle, would you? Scare yourself sometime and actually read the ingredient lists for popular cereals. The most prevalent ingredient is detailed first, and the list proceeds from there. If sugar appears in the top five, don't buy it!

You might as well sit your little tyke down and put 5 tablespoons of sugar in a bowl and let him dig in. The American Dietetic Association recommends no more than 6 grams of sugar per serving. My advice is to try to lower that even more.

A classic marketing ploy is flooding a high-sugar cereal with vitamins and fiber. You can always get the vitamins and fiber you need from non-sugary sources, so don't be bamboozled by a cereal box screaming about its healthy daily vitamin supply. In addition, make sure the saturated fat content is minimal (< 1 gram per serving). There are many cereals that contain no saturated fats, so this should be your standard. With the multiplicity of choices there is no logical reason for picking a high-sugar (> 6 grams per serving) or a high saturated fat (any at all) cereal. Also, whole grain is much more preferred than bleached flour, wheat, rice, corn, or barley.

A Sugar Comparison

The sugar content in a 50-gram serving of popular cereals and candies:

Sugar Crisp cereal	26.6g
Kit Kat bar	26.19g
Snickers bar	25.42g
Nesquik cereal	23.3g
Froot Loops	22.5g
Cocoa Puffs	22.2g
Trix	21.6g
Frosted Cheerios	21.6g
Lucky Charms	21.6g
Frosted Flakes	12.1g
Rice Krispies	5.35g

Source: company reports

Basically, the best way to select a cereal is the rule of 3s. Each serving must contain less than 3 grams of fat, at least 3 grams of fiber, and less than 2 x 3 (6) grams of sugar.

ARTIFICIAL SWEETENERS

You can't discuss cereal without mentioning the ubiquitous artificial sweeteners. And it is not just cereals anymore. These substances show up in anything from drinks to desserts. Realistically, most cereals are already laden with so much sugar that adding more is like putting pancake syrup on a birthday cake, yet we persist in using both table sugar (sucrose) and a variety of artificial sweeteners to further seal our doom and thrill our taste buds.

Artificial sweeteners or sugar substitutes have been with us for over fifty years, and their use is surrounded with confusion and controversy. Many see them as a viable, calorie-free option to make food more pleasurable, whereas others view them as carcinogenic poisons. I suspect the truth lies somewhere between those extremes, as is often the case. Some common sugar substitutes available today are aspartame (NutraSweet, Equal), acesulfame potassium (Sweet One, Sunett), sucralose (Splenda), and neotame. Many food products contain sugar alcohols such as sorbitol and mannitol and, although they contain calories, they don't elevate the blood sugar as much as table sugar.

The main advantage bestowed on artificial sweeteners is that they neither contain calories nor raise the blood sugar level. This is a good thing, right? Not necessarily. From the outset these products have come under scrutiny by health agencies for potential side effects. In 1969 the U.S. Food and Drug Administration (FDA) banned cyclamate, an early artificial sweetener, because of a possible link to bladder cancer. Today the most prolific substitute—and the most controversial—is aspartame.

What about the plethora of breakfast bars promising a nutritional start to the day? They are little more than glorified candy bars marketed as a breakfast substitute. If you routinely feed your child a Snickers bar for breakfast, then these may be a suitable substitute.

Aspartame was approved in 1981 by the FDA after numerous tests showed that it did not cause cancer or other adverse effects in laboratory animals. Questions regarding the safety of aspartame were renewed by a 1996 report suggesting that an increase in the number of people with brain tumors between 1975 and 1992 might be associated with the introduction and use of this sweetener in the United States. However, an analysis of then-current National Cancer Institute statistics showed that the overall incidents of brain cancers began to rise in 1973, eight years prior to the approval of aspartame, and continued to rise until 1985. Moreover, increases in overall brain cancer incidents occurred primarily in people age seventy and older, a group that was not exposed to the highest doses of aspartame since its introduction. These data do not establish a clear link between the consumption of aspartame and the development of brain tumors.[1]

Headaches are probably the most common side effect attributed to aspartame use, but some anecdotal reports list panic attacks, mood changes, visual hallucinations, manic episodes, dizziness, nervousness, memory impairment, nausea, temper outbursts, and depression. None of these conditions has been rigorously proven to be caused by aspartame. Because of its ubiquitous nature, parents must be vigilant in their children's overall aspartame consumption. For example, a two-year-old drinking one 12-ounce diet soda can get the maximum recommended intake of aspartame in that alone. Go back to the basic rule of nutrition: everything in moderation. There are some people who are exquisitely sensitive to some chemicals, and this may be magnified in children because of their lower body weight.

The take-home point is to avoid excessive use of products that are heavily sweetened with aspartame (no six diet sodas a day!) or other artificial sweeteners. What is healthy to use as a sweetener when needed? Good old table sugar and honey, in moderation. None of any of these things will make you grow two heads or turn your skin purple, but you have to exercise restraint and uncommon sense. Go ahead and sprinkle a little sugar on their whole-grain cereal, or mix some honey on your kids' oatmeal, but do it in limited amounts.

Healthy and Quick Breakfast Ideas

Fruit Smoothies. My kids love these, and they take five minutes to make. Take one or a combination of fruits your kids like, mix in some ice and water, and you can even add a tablespoon of protein powder (they will never know). Put it all in a blender, let it fly, and they get a healthy, fiber-filled, nutritious, simple, quick breakfast. The night before you can even put the ingredients in separate containers and just pop them into the blender first thing in the morning to save even more time.

Low-Fat Yogurt With Nuts. Take the yogurt out of the cup and put it in a bowl with nuts or berries (again, you can do this the night before). Have the kids help prepare the dish, as this gives them ownership and begins the process of education by participation.

Oatmeal or Cream of Wheat. This is a longtime staple because it is healthy. Put some honey on top and you have a delightful combination that provides fuel for the day. Watch out for some oatmeal products that have a number of additives that increase the sugar and fat content.

And now some weird but effective suggestions from *www.kidshealth.org*:
Banana Dog. Peanut butter, a banana, and raisins in a long whole-grain bun.
Breakfast Taco. Shredded low-fat cheese on a tortilla, folded in half and microwaved; top with salsa.
Country Cottage Cheese. Apple butter mixed with cottage cheese.
Fruit and Cream Cheese Sandwich. Use strawberries or other fresh fruit.

LUNCHABLES

Dr. Albert Goldberg writes in his fabulous book *Feed Your Child Right*: "What is the typical teenage lunch or snack? A Big Mac, French fries, and a chocolate shake provide 1000 calories, with 31 grams of fat . . . 50% of these calories are from fat! . . . In addition, the Big Mac has 960 milligrams of sodium, and that doesn't include what is on the French fries. There is negligible fiber and excess sugar. Many school cafeteria lunches are as bad, or worse."[2]

Children and teens find themselves in unique situations for lunch during the school year. Often they are given very limited choices, and many of those choices are devastatingly bad. Many of the public school lunch programs in this country are sorely lacking in quality and variety. I understand the limitations of budget and bureaucracy, but these are the same people who categorized ketchup as a vegetable. In an attempt to circumvent the monetary crises in schools, certain creative minds have enlisted the help of corporate America. The result is that our kids are being bombarded with propaganda (they call it education)—sponsored, endorsed, and encouraged by local school boards.

> "Their foods tend to be at the bottom of the barrel in terms of healthy nutrition."
>
> —Dr. Walter Willett, head of the Department of Nutrition at the Harvard School of Public Health, commenting on school lunch programs

"Today the nation's fast food chains are marketing their products in public schools through conventional ad campaigns, classroom teaching materials, and lunchroom franchises, as well as a number of unorthodox means," writes Eric Schlosser in *Fast Food Nation*.[3] The American School Food Service Association estimates that about

30 percent of public high schools in the United States offer branded fast food (McDonald's, Burger King, Pizza Hut, Domino's, Taco Bell, etc.).[4]

The rationale for this nutritional abomination ranges from "we need the money" to "we want the kids to see us as cool and not institutional." These administrators are trying to overcome their budget woes and lack of leadership on the backs of your kids. Your children are being dragged into the obesity abyss for the sake of corporate profits. The irresponsible school boards then compound the problem by eliminating physical education programs, thus condemning a preponderance of children to portliness. A step in the right direction came in 2006 when the nation's largest beverage distributors agreed to stop selling non-diet sodas to most public schools. This agreement also included stocking vending machines with more bottled water, unsweetened fruit juices, and low-fat milk—all in smaller portions. Even so, diet drinks still contain loads of sodium and caffeine.

So what can be done to help our kids during the approximately 150 days a year they are in school? First, examine your own school system's lunch program. Visit and eat there once or twice. Ask to see a weekly menu. Find out if any fast-food establishments have invaded the lunchroom. Determine who sets the menus and what guidelines they use. All this could be done in one afternoon, and I guarantee that you will understand more in that afternoon than most parents ever know. If what you discover is frightening, either work within the system to change things, or commit to send your child to school with a healthier lunch. This is a great opportunity to teach children and teens about healthy choices. In some situations, children do have a choice of the food they eat at school, and some of the choices are surprisingly healthy. If your kids are aware of what is good, they are at least slightly more apt to choose wisely. Realistically, teens will probably choose whatever tastes best and what their peers are eating. Who knows, they may actually enjoy being trendsetters or rebels and convince their friends to join them in their quest for health. Some kids are becoming activists and leading the fight to restore school lunchrooms to healthy environments. What a great way to channel their teenage rebellion!

You can't discuss adolescent nutrition without addressing the issue of "liquid candy," otherwise known as drinks, sodas, and a variety of readily available beverages. Changing behaviors in this one area can significantly alter your child's health both now and in the future. The Center for Science in the Public Interest estimates that the average teenager derives 9 to 10 percent of his or her daily calorie intake from soft drinks. The average child will consume four to five cans of soda a day—and with each can having the equivalent of ten teaspoons of sugar, you can easily understand why we are facing an epidemic of childhood obesity and diabetes.

If you want to impress your teen, sit her down at breakfast, take out a cereal bowl, and proceed to dump in 40 teaspoons of sugar. This dramatically demonstrates what she may be putting into her body each day solely from drinks.

> An extra can of soda a day can pile on fifteen pounds in a year.
> Source: *American Journal of Clinical Nutrition,* August 2006

And that is just the sugar! Some beverages contain enough caffeine to arouse a moose, let alone a seventy-five-pound fifth-grader. As discussed earlier, even diet drinks are laden with sodium, artificial sweeteners, and sometimes caffeine. I don't even need to mention the problems with such "energy" drinks like Red Bull and Full Throttle—the names say it all. These drinks are little more than a delivery system for caffeine and sugar.

This travesty is not limited to teens. Michael Jacobson, author of *Liquid Candy*, reports, "Pepsi, Dr Pepper, and Seven-Up encourage feeding soft drinks to babies by licensing their logos to a major maker of baby bottles, Munchkin Bottling, Inc." Parents have to wake up and realize their kids are being indoctrinated into a destructive lifestyle of obesity, diabetes, heart disease, osteoporosis, and premature death.

So what are some healthy options for lunches and drinks? When it comes to beverages, nothing is as healthy and vital as water. For kids and adults alike, water is what God designed us to consume. Use lemon, lime, or other fresh fruit to flavor the water. Keep water bottles in the car, in backpacks, and in the fridge. Sales of bottled water to both kids and adults have skyrocketed in the last few years because it has become cool to drink. Hey, whatever works! Check the labels on the abundant "flavored" waters to make sure they are not filled with artificial sweeteners and other nutritionally hollow substances. Unsweetened fruit juices are generally healthy and have an abundance of vitamins and nutrients. It is important to distinguish fresh, pure fruit juice from the imitators marketed to kids. Read the labels! Skim milk contains calcium and other minerals and is generally recognized as a healthy drink, in spite of some radical vegetarians' claims of hormone contamination. (The pasteurization process removes any of these harmful substances.) Eight ounces of vegetable juice has 2 grams of fiber, is very low in sugar, and has only 50 calories. And don't forget about fresh fruit smoothies!

Healthy Lunch Options

* Vegetarian or lean meat hamburgers

* Grilled cheese sandwiches with non-fat cheese

* Soy ravioli

* Fat-free yogurt

* Fruit salads

* Lean turkey sandwich with non-fat mayonnaise and whole-wheat bread

* Low-fat bean burrito

* Chili dog using soy dogs and non-fat chili

* Spaghetti with low-fat tomato meat sauce

* Low-fat yogurt and granola mix

Dr. Albert Goldberg, author and nutritionist, lists ten healthy foods that can be incorporated in lunches in virtually any situation: sweet potatoes, whole-grain bread, broccoli, strawberries, beans, cantaloupe, spinach and kale, oranges, oatmeal, and skim milk.[5] Be creative, think abnormally!

A FAMILY BANQUET

I have already pointed out the importance of a family eating together. It is vital that you make heroic attempts to corral the family several times a week for meals; often the evening meal is the most practical time to accomplish this. Here is where you practice what you preach, and kids learn by what they observe. The same principles apply to this meal as all others, yet consciously expunge convention and purposely reduce the calorie content of the evening meal. As has been shown, most American households actually consume the greatest number of calories at night. Simply decreasing the total calories of the evening meal can help a person's weight, sleep, energy level, and mood. Dinner is a great time to guarantee that adequate vitamins and minerals are ingested—especially if you can't control what your kids (or spouse) eats at lunch.

EATING OUT

Eating out is an important part of daily life in the United States, and the trend (an expensive one) continues to grow unabated. According to the National Restaurant Association, each American, eight years and older, ate an average of 4.3 commercially prepared meals per week in 1998, up from 3.9 meals just five years earlier. If going to a restaurant is the only way to coerce the family to eat together regularly, at least attempt to make the experience beneficial socially and nutritionally by following some simple suggestions from the American Heart Association:

- Ask the server to make substitutions like having steamed vegetables instead of French fries.

- Pick lean meat, fish, or skinless chicken.

- Make sure your entrée is broiled, baked, grilled, steamed, or poached instead of fried.

- Order vegetable side dishes and ask that any sauces or butter be left off.

- Ask for low-calorie salad dressing or a lemon to squeeze on your salad instead of dressing.

- Ask for baked, boiled, or roasted potatoes instead of fried—and ask for them without the butter and sour cream.

- Order fresh fruit or fruit sorbet in place of cake, pie, or ice-cream desserts.

- Ask about low-fat or fat-free choices.

The key to getting healthy food when eating out is to be bold and ask. Your family deserves it!

In addition, realize that portions in restaurants are generally too large. Don't admonish the kids to clean their plate, or they may explode! Stay away from all-you-can-eat food troughs and buffets. These may seem like good values economically, but you will physically pay dearly from the chronic gorging. If the restaurant traditionally offers bread before the meal, either ask your server not to bring it or to bring it with the meal itself. Not grazing before the meal can eliminate a tremendous number of unhealthy calories.

These are only guidelines. Is it okay to occasionally eat bread before a meal? Of course! Is it ever all right to have a dessert? Sure, if you have the discipline to limit how much you eat and the number of times you order dessert. Eating out can be a special treat for the whole family, but don't use it as an excuse for gluttony.

—— FAT-PROOF POINTERS ——

The adolescent and teen years are absolutely critical in the overall plan to fat-proof your family.

Don't use the term *diet* with children or adolescents; to them that will imply restriction and generally elicit rebellion.

With your children, as with you, amounts matter, variety is key, exercise is mandatory, and modeling is the best teaching device.

At the end of the day, fat-proofing your family is about teaching and learning.

Breakfast (break the fast) is the cornerstone in building a healthy, nutritional lifestyle for your child.

Find out if any fast-food establishments have invaded your school's lunchroom.

If your kids are aware of what is good, they are at least slightly more apt to choose wisely.

If going to a restaurant is the only way to coerce the family to eat together regularly, at least attempt to make the experience beneficial socially and nutritionally.

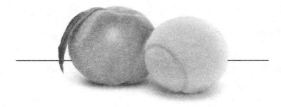

WEIGHT LOSS

IT'S **NOT THE PROBLEM** YOU THINK IT IS!

"Okay, Susan, today we start! This is the beginning of the battle of the bulge!" Blanca continued, "I am going to lose twenty pounds before my class reunion or I am going with a bag over my head!"

Susan understood the desperation in Blanca's voice. She wanted to drop a few pounds herself.

"Blanca, we have to stick together; this will be like Alcoholics Anonymous. I'll call you if I have a craving for fried chicken and you call me for a chocolate sneak attack. Together we stand, divided we get fatter!"

Blanca felt stronger and lighter already. "And one more thing, Susan. I signed us both up at that new Curves on Wheeler Avenue. We can have our own personal trainers!"

"You did what?!" Susan said incredulously. "Are you talking about me sweating? A gym with shorts and cellulite all over and guys lifting twenty million pounds watching me struggle with a toothpick? No way, no ma'am, no how!"

Blanca was ready for her response. "I thought you'd react like that, but this place is a women-only club and it's even cheaper than that weird abdominal thing you bought on the Shopping Network last year."

"Well, that sounds a bit better, and I do want to lose the weight. Maybe I'll give it a try and see," Susan said. "Besides, I sold that abdominal thing on eBay last month."

IT'S NOT WEIGHT LOSS, IT'S FAT GAIN!

Three of the most common medical complaints of parents are: "I'm overweight"; "I have no energy"; and "My sex drive has driven off!" It seems that the obvious solution to all three problems would be to figure out how to have energetic, aerobic, fat-burning sex! But if that is physically impossible or psychologically unimaginable, here is some practical advice on one of those problems, weight loss.

If you are looking for a quick fix, look elsewhere. It should be obvious by now that miracle diets and amazing new pills are not the answer. The keys to this "tough love" fat-loss program are knowledge, dedication, and perseverance. Dr. Colin Campbell writes, "Keeping body weight off is a long term lifestyle choice. Gimmicks that produce impressively large, quick weight losses don't work in the long term."[1] And it is not just parents that are interested in fat control. As you know by now, the family has to be a part of the equation in any lasting program to control weight and get fit. The principles of fat freedom apply to all members of the family. Involve everyone if lasting success is to be achieved. So buckle your belts and let's get started on the last fat-control regimen you will ever need.

This chapter is designed for the person who is interested in losing five to fifty pounds of fat. Even though some minor changes apply, this advice is applicable to both children and adults. Although many of the principles still apply, this is not for the very obese person with multiple medical problems. The excessively obese guy or gal should only work under the care of a trained bariatrician (weight loss physician).

Another important caveat at the outset: When I use the term *weight loss,* I really mean *fat* loss (though you may have already surmised that). You want to lose body fat to be fit. All these suggestions are linked to reducing your percent body fat, not losing muscle or lean mass. And actually, the problem is not losing weight. Everyone can lose weight. We all do it . . . and do it . . . and do it. *Losing weight* is actually relatively easy. What we all need is a way to lose the fat . . . and not regain it! The problem is *gaining fat*! Remember, it is not about losing, but about winning the battle with your body to produce a lean, mean, fat-burning machine!

Talk to most overweight persons and they will say unapologetically that they realize they are jeopardizing their health. Even those who are comfortable with their weight psychologically admit they would be physically healthier if they lost a few pounds. Amy Joy Lanou, nutrition director of the Physicians Committee for Responsible Medicine, writes, "In the realm of nutrition, we need a hearty helping of tough love. Let's end our dysfunctional love affair with greasy burgers and artery clogging chicken nuggets. Instead we will embark on a rewarding long-term relationship with meals full of fruits, vegetables, legumes and whole grains."[2]

> **Did You Know?**
>
> Leptin (from the Greek word *leptos*, meaning thin) is a hormone that plays a key role in regulating energy intake and energy expenditure, including the regulation of appetite and metabolism. Binding of leptin to the hypothalamus signals to the brain that the body has had enough to eat—a sensation of satiety. A tremendous amount of interest is being directed at leptin, so expect to hear more about it soon as a possible tool for combating obesity.

Since the explosion of knowledge gained by mapping the human genome, there has been great speculation that being overweight is more of a genetic problem than one of environment; the classic "nature vs. nurture" argument. The unpopular reality is only a small percentage of overweight individuals actually have a metabolic syndrome that contributes to their excess poundage. While this is true, there is mounting evidence that some people's genes do make them more predisposed to excessive weight gain. In other words, given similar food intake, some folks will put on weight whereas others might not.

The recent discovery of the fat-regulating hormone leptin has fueled speculation that a physiological breakthrough in the treatment of obesity is on the horizon. Will it be possible for you to simply replace a missing hormone someday and achieve normal weight? Maybe. There are already documented cases where this has been accomplished in animals, but scientists are years away from developing a safe and effective tool. Even so, this would not be a panacea, as it would only be helpful in those who lack the missing hormone. Nevertheless, there is mounting evidence that *marked* obesity is a disease rather than a lack of willpower. We already know that the drive to eat is regulated in the hypothalamus, a small organ below the brain, so it may be that a malfunction in that organ could trigger behavior that results in severe obesity. To be sure, I am speaking here about folks who are very obese (BMI > 34), not those of you who need to lose ten or twenty pounds. Jeffrey Friedman writes in *Science* magazine, "Obesity is not a personal failing. In trying to lose weight, the obese are fighting a difficult battle. It is a battle against biology, a battle that only the intrepid take on and one in which only a few prevail."[3] Fat cells are actually very active systems shooting out a myriad of chemical messengers that inevitably produce a vicious cycle; the fatter you get, the more chemicals are produced by your own body to keep you that way! For the mildly overweight person (BMI 25–29), the key is moderate fat loss to block this process.

Simple math can tell you the calorie content of any food if you know the amount of protein, fat, and carbohydrate in the food. You simply multiply the number of grams by the number of calories in a gram of that food component. For example, if a serving of fries (about twenty fries—not super-sized!) has 16 grams of fat, 144 calories are from fat. That's 16 grams × 9 calories per gram.

As I have indicated, the solution to routine weight loss is simple, uncommonly common, and it works for both individuals and families. It is not hype; it is not "new"; it is not a "secret." It is the *only* fat-loss regimen that has been rigorously tested and survives intact today because it is based on valid science, not marketing. So what do you have to do to lose weight? Actually, a better question is, what do you have to do to lose extra body fat? You will see the difference shortly.

WEIGHT LOSS 101

The first step to fat control is to honestly examine what you are currently eating, and the second step is to reduce it! If you weren't eating too much, you wouldn't be in the fix you are in.

Don't let anyone fool you. Total calories matter, and they matter a great deal. Some diet plans state that the total calories consumed are not as important as the kind of calories. There is a grain of truth to that, but it mainly pertains to which calories are burned and which are stored. If you eat 800 calories of protein and 800 calories of fat, some of both will be converted to body fat if they are not burned up by activity or metabolism. A calorie by any other name is still a calorie, regardless of the source.

A calorie is simply a measure of energy generated when a substance is metabolized. (Here *calorie* actually represents 1 kilocalorie, but to avoid confusion, I will continue to use the term calorie.) A gram of protein yields 4 calories when it is burned. A gram of carbohydrate yields 4 calories when it is metabolized, and a gram of fat yields 9 calories when it is consumed. (By the way, a gram of alcohol yields 7 calories when consumed.) To summarize:

Source of Energy	Calories per Gram
Fat	9
Carbohydrate	4
Protein	4

It is easy to see that, gram for gram, fat is a great concentrated source of energy; energy that you have to expend or it will stay with you in the form of love handles and jelly bellies.

The source of the calories does not change the energy content. A gram of protein from Bessie the cow will yield the same energy as a gram of protein from Sally soybean, assuming it is completely metabolized. There is no question that the source and kind of nutrient will have different effects on things like cholesterol synthesis, but the calories remain the same. Therefore, a recommendation to decrease your calorie intake means decrease the *total* intake of calories, regardless of the source. This doesn't mean that you should live on only one source of calories (i.e., eating protein bars morning, noon, and night), because there is more to nutrition than just calories.

There has to be a balance of nutrients, vitamins, minerals, and water to keep our bodies functioning. So the challenge is to keep the calorie content reasonable while getting a balance of nutrients. Dr. Andrew Weil writes in his wonderful book *Eating Well for Optimum Health,* "In losing weight you should continue to eat about 50–60% calories as carbohydrate, 30% as fat and 10–20% as protein, but you must reduce the amount you eat, both by decreasing the size of the portions and by cutting down on the snacking, especially the kind of unconscious snacking that many people do as a nervous habit."[4] Many bariatricians (physicians with special training in weight control) embrace this practice of a "balanced deficit lifestyle" as a tool for fat loss.

> For decades, studies have shown a direct link between calorie restriction and longevity. In other words, decreasing your calorie intake (to a point) seems to reduce the processes that contribute to aging and morbidity. Most of this research is the proverbial white rat studies, so it would be unfair to draw direct conclusions for humans, but the data does look promising that decreasing your total calorie intake will not only help you lose weight, but will also prolong your life.

TAKING INVENTORY

To risk redundancy, the first step in your quest for weight control is being very aware of what you eat; then reduce it! This is an absolute necessity. It is similar to setting a budget for your family; the first step is finding out where you are currently spending money. Likewise, in limiting calories, you start by assessing where the calories currently originate.

Your first task is to take three days of the week, preferably a Thursday, Friday, and Saturday (to see both weekday and weekend eating habits), and write down every piece of food, drink, or snack that passes your lips. This information will be used to determine how many calories you and your family are consuming. Also note the mode of preparation (baked, fried, steamed, etc.) for food items. How a meal is prepared can often add more calories than the actual food itself. It should be obvious that a plate of fried chicken is a bit more destructive for your coronary arteries than a plate of broiled chicken.

Engage the family in this activity. Try to make it a game, and give a prize to the family member with the most complete record. (You can help the younger kids do this; what a great lesson for them also!) Include the time of the day and amounts in your food "diary." Some estimates are dangerous at this stage because most studies indicate that you will underestimate your consumption by 30 to 40 percent, so try to be as accurate as possible here. A simple yet accurate tool is the "hand method":

Helpful things to note in a food diary:

- How much (in grams or servings)
- What kind (protein, fat, carb)
- Where (home, office, car)
- With whom (alone or family)
- Time (morning, night)
- Mood (depressed, sad, top-of-the-world, etc.)
- Activity (what you are doing while eating)

- One closed fist = one cup of beverage
- Two cupped hands = cup of flaky cereal, salad, soup, or one ounce of chips
- Two thumbs up = one tablespoon of peanut butter, salad dressing, cream cheese, margarine
- One thumb up = one ounce of cheese
- One cupped hand = half cup of pasta, rice, cut fruit, berries; one ounce of nuts
- Palm of hand = three ounces of cooked meat or fish

I said at the outset this was no easy fix. This is the first test of your commitment. You have to become painfully aware of your present habits. Don't try to change your normal eating style during this time. Don't begin by lying to yourself. Once you have done this for three days, stop crying, and then analyze the total calorie content of each day by breaking it down into calories per meal. This is relatively easy with the food labeling and serving size guidelines. There are several resources available to calculate the calorie content of most foods.

For nutrient data ...

Web sites

nutrition.gov

nutritiondata.com

nal.usda.gov/fnic/foodcomp/search/

calorieking.com/foods

fda.gov

foodfileonline.com

Books

Corinne Netzer's *Complete Book of Food Counts*

The Calorie King Calorie, Fat & Carbohydrate Counter by Allan Borushek

Devices and software

dietorganizer.com

fitday.com

caloriecountingsoftware.com

Most nutritionists recommend 1,700 to 2,500 calories a day for active adults. The Food and Nutrition Board of the National Research Council has suggested an intake of 2,000 calories a day for women performing light work between the ages of twenty-three and fifty. Don't get confused. This is not to say you can consume 2,000 calories of just anything and stay healthy. There has to be a balance. A reasonable and sustainable mix is 50 percent low-glycemic carbohydrates, 30 percent protein, and 20 percent mostly mono- and polyunsaturated fats. That is a broad range, so you can see from the outset that these calculations must be individualized to be useful. As we shall see, the operative word in this recommendation is *active* adults. Note that these are general recommendations. Your particular need will vary with your fitness level, current weight, and goals.

Age	Average Calorie Needs Each Day
0–5 months	650
5–12 months	850
1–3 years	1300
4–6 years	1800
7–10 years	2000

Boys	Average Calorie Needs Each Day
11–14 years	2500
15–18 years	3000
Girls	**Average Calorie Needs Each Day**
11–14 years	2200
15–18 years	2200

Source: Vincent Iannelli, MD, F.A.A.P., President, Keep Kids Healthy, LLC, Member American Academy of Pediatrics

One reason people fail in dieting is because they get sick of counting calories. It becomes tedious and eventually dominates their life. They don't like the restrictions. The cold, hard reality is that there is no other way . . . initially. It becomes much less of a burden once you adopt the habit of estimating the calorie content of meals. With practice, you will be able to look at a plate of food and get a reasonable estimate of the calorie content; it just takes some effort and practice. Think of the amount of time you spend on watching TV each day (or any preferred distraction). Isn't it worth taking at least some of that brain-numbing time and devoting it to learning how to estimate calories?

If you find yourself consuming 3,000 calories a day and are twenty pounds overweight, then to lose weight you obviously have to reduce your calorie intake. The secret is to do it over time. Jumping into an 800-calorie-per-day diet (remember, we are using *diet* as a noun, not a verb) will make you lose weight quickly, but you will feel terrible, become cranky, and try to run over small dogs with your car. This type of radical calorie restriction is neither healthy nor productive over the long haul. What you should be targeting is *sustainable* fat loss and maintenance that becomes a way of life. A F-A-D diet really means *f*eeling *a*wful *d*aily.

SLOW CHANGES

Studies indicate the majority of us are consuming more calories now than ever before. This has to stop. Do it gradually. Take small steps to facilitate success. Buy smaller packages and use smaller plates. If you are currently eating 2,500 calories a day, don't worry about calculations, just reduce your intake the first week by 10 percent (250 calories a day). This may be as simple as two fewer sodas a day. On week number two, drop your intake by another 10 percent. After that, go through the calorie calculations for the desired weight loss and adjust your intake accordingly.

A common question is, "How many calories do I need every day to maintain and not gain?" This amount will vary depending on your height, body type, and most important, your exercise habits. A simple formula utilizes a term called the basal metabolic rate

> Experts say perseverance and hard work—not quick fixes—are key to losing and keeping off weight. Shoot for one to two pounds a week. Any more may result in losing muscle instead of fat.

(BMR). Your BMR is the energy used (measured in calories) by your body to perform basic functions, including internal energy expenditure, breathing, and body temperature regulation. It is the number of calories your body would expend if you laid on the couch and watched reruns of *Everybody Loves Raymond* every day.

A simple tool for calculating your BMR is:

Body weight in pounds × 13.5 (calories/lb) = _____

This number gives you an estimate as to what it takes (in calories) to keep you functioning at a basic level. Keep in mind this is an estimate, as many of the factors listed above can vary over time, thus changing the calculation. Since you are not interested in writing research papers, this simplified calculation will suffice. The most important number is not your BMR at your present weight, but what it will be at your target weight. (Remember from chapter 1, you can get an idea of a healthy target weight from the BMI table.)

The number of calories you need depends on many different factors such as your age, health, body type and size, and your activity. Some very active persons are able to eat large amounts of food and not gain weight, while those who are less active do gain weight. People who have rounded, soft body types called endomorphs seem to gain weight more easily than those who have slender, wiry body types called ectomorphs. Those who gain weight just looking at food are called Pillsbury Doughmorphs.

WHAT YOU NEED

Another way to find out how many calories you need to maintain your present weight is to multiply the amount of energy you use times your weight. If you are inactive, multiply by 14 to 16 calories; if you're moderately active, multiply by 16 to 18 calories; and if you're very active, multiply your weight in pounds by 18 to 20 calories. For example, an inactive woman weighing 120 pounds would multiply 120 by 14, which would equal 1,680. This is the amount of calories she would need each day to maintain her present weight, again a rough estimate of her BMR.

If you want to lose fat, you have to burn more calories (mainly through exercise) than you take in. One pound of body fat represents 3,500 calories. In order to gain one pound, you must eat 3,500 calories more than your body needs. Sounds tough, but I suspect we all can climb that mountain! Therefore, in order to lose a pound of body fat, you must eat less and burn off a total of 3,500 calories in excess of your basic metabolic needs. If you reduce your caloric intake by 500 calories a day for a week, the projected loss in body fat would be one pound. I am assuming, for simplicity, that all the weight loss is fat. Realistically this is not the case, especially in non-exercisers. Keep in mind, this is reducing the calories required to maintain your current weight, if your weight is stable.

If you are putting on pounds with your present eating habits, then basing anything on your current weight is worthless. However, if your weight is stable, then using your current weight to calculate your current BMR is meaningful. If your BMR is 2,000 calories, but you are currently eating 3,000 calories a day, simply eating 2,500 calories a day (reducing your daily intake by 500) will not help much if that is all you do. You have to either bring in less than required to maintain current weight, or burn off more, or both. Remember that you are looking at pounds of actual body fat loss, not just changes in body weight, and this comes only from changing your body chemistry through exercise. Initial weight loss, for many, is mostly water. In fact, it is reasonable to say that any loss in the first two weeks of almost any diet is largely fluid.

THERE'S SOMETHING ABOUT MARY

Let's take a practical example and work through a calculation of calories needed for a slow, sustainable weight loss. Mary is thirty-five and beginning to notice that she is putting on a few pounds. She is five feet four and weighs 160 pounds. She would like to lose ten pounds. With her current eating habits her weight has stabilized. She will have to decrease her calorie intake (from her BMR) by 35,000 calories to achieve this (3,500 calories per pound X 10 pounds to lose). At her target weight, if Mary is not exercising, her BMR (the number of calories to maintain her target weight) is 2,025 calories (150 pounds [her target weight] × 13.5). So she needs to consume about 2,000 calories per day (rounding makes it easier) to maintain her weight at 150. But she needs to get there first.

After Mary did her food diary she found out she was currently consuming about 3,000 calories a day. At her current weight, her BMR is 2,160 (160 [current weight] × 13.5), so you can see all that extra is going to be stored if it is not used. She can take this 2,160 and reduce it by 200 calories a day, and after about six months she will have decreased her total intake the 35,000 calories she needed to lose the weight. Step number one then is to reduce her current intake (3,000 calories/day) to her calculated BMR for her target weight (2,160). Once Mary does this over time, then she can work on further calorie reduction. This time frame for weight loss can be dramatically shortened by exercise and a greater calorie restriction. Say she decreases her calories to 1,860 a day (very realistic!) and walks for thirty minutes a day. The time frame for losing the weight now drops to about two months! This is not only healthier than a more rapid weight loss, but it is sustainable. You can live this way and not feel like you are starved all the time. Reducing calories in about 10- to 20-percent increments are tolerable and sustainable.

To simplify things, Mary just needs to decrease her calorie intake 25 percent (while eating a diet balanced at 50 percent low-glycemic carbohydrates, 30 percent protein, and 20 percent fat) and exercise thirty minutes a day, and over time, the weight will come off.

Some of you may be thinking, *All those calculations make my head hurt. I'll never keep this up.* Don't be put off by the numbers. I included these calculations solely for my obsessive brethren. The principle is simple. Decrease the amount of calories you are eating now, and begin an exercise program with the whole family. The steps are simple: (1) determine what you are currently eating, (2) decrease your total calorie intake in slow, deliberate increments [10 to 15 percent every two weeks] until you reach a level that will maintain your desired weight, and (3) exercise to burn off excess calories.

"Using a tape measure, you can record the circumference of different areas of the body. This allows you to see at an instant when you're losing weight, gaining, or staying the same. Tape measurements are good when you're just starting out because you'll see a definite improvement within the first six weeks. Clothes will fit better and you'll see the numbers gradually get smaller and smaller."

—Michelle Silence, MA, *www.thedietchannel.com*

PATIENCE, PERSISTENCE, AND PREDICTABLE RESULTS

Weight loss may vary for several reasons. This is where your will is going to be tested. The two most dangerous potholes on the path to establishing a healthy eating regimen are not seeing quick results and hitting a plateau. Daily changes in body fluid also affect your weight. Just because you weigh one pound more in the evening than you weighed that morning doesn't mean that you've gained one pound of body fat. Fluctuations that are that rapid are almost always fluid. Likewise, women may see rather dramatic weight changes from water retention depending on where they are in their cycle. I'm lucky, my body just retains doughnuts!

Sustainable weight loss is accomplished slowly. It is physiologically impossible to lose five pounds of body fat in forty-eight hours, unless you visit a plastic surgeon. If you drop that in weight, it is always mostly fluid, and inevitably will come right back. Patience and persistence breeds long-term success. Calvin Coolidge said, "Nothing in this world can take the place of persistence. Talent will not; nothing is more common than unsuccessful men with talent. Genius will not; unrewarded genius is almost a proverb. Education will not; the world is full of educated derelicts."

Set a reasonable target of two to three pounds of body fat every two weeks. Our goal is fitness, not necessarily thinness. The best way to break through a plateau in weight loss is to increase your exercise time or intensity. In most cases, either starting an exercise program or ratcheting up a current regimen gets you past those nagging last few pounds.

Eat a variety of foods, keeping the 50 percent low-glycemic carbohydrate, 30 percent protein, and 20 percent fat ratio in mind. Most of the restriction diets (Atkins, South Beach, etc.) are so constraining that only the most obsessive person can actually make it a lifestyle. Variety is the key to long-term compliance. The reality is that you must eat balanced, nutritious meals, but in smaller portions. Take each day as a unit. If you eat more for breakfast, cut back a little at dinner. If the math is too intimidating or confusing, ask a dietitian to calculate how many calories you need to eat in a day for sustainable weight loss. Every hospital has dietitians on staff that can do a brief individual consultation and supply you with a target calorie goal.

I realize this sounds almost absurd in its simplicity, yet if you break down any successful diet plan to its most basic constituents, you will find calorie restriction as a bedrock principle. Even fad diets work temporarily because you end up eating fewer total calories.

FASTING FOR FUN AND PROFIT

Since we are focusing on intake, I want to address a topic that many in the Christian community ask about: fasting. The practice of fasting for both religious and health reasons is an ancient one. Historical documents report that Socrates, Plato, Pythagoras, and Hippocrates all recommended fasting for various medical conditions. Almost every major religion of the twenty-first century utilizes fasting in some form in their rituals and worship. Fasting is an important event in both Old and New Testament teachings.

Jesus fasted forty days in the desert prior to his public ministry, and there are numerous examples of Jesus and his followers fasting in the Gospels. "And when you fast, don't make it obvious, as the hypocrites do, who try to look pale and disheveled so people will admire them for their fasting. I assure you, that is the only reward they will ever get. But when you fast, comb your hair

> Hippocrates, the father of medicine, used fasting to combat disease 2,400 years ago. The ancient Ayurvedic healers of the Hindu religion prescribed fasting weekly for a healthy digestive system. Most nationalities, religions, and languages have a tradition of fasting handed down from their ancestors.
>
> Source: Dr. Rex Russell, in *What the Bible Says About Healthy Living*

and wash your face. Then no one will suspect you are fasting, except your Father, who knows what you do in secret. And your Father, who knows all secrets, will reward you" (Matthew 6:16–18).

In this context, fasting is primarily a religious practice. It is not practiced as a weight loss tool. The primary focus of this type of fasting is on spiritual renewal and worship.

Some types of fasting have been used in certain weight loss regimens, especially those with a spiritual foundation. Dr. Joel Fuhrman, a national expert on therapeutic fasting, cautions, "If a person is unwilling or unable to make permanent changes in the diet and follow a healthy eating plan before and after the fast, there is really no point in fasting."[5]

There are as many variations on fasting as there are people participating in them. Some restrict meat, whereas others restrict all foods. Some include juices and other drinks, while some use only water. Fasting solely for weight loss is obviously not a sustainable method. It is like a swat team; a quick in and a quick out. It accomplishes the short-term goal, but that level of intensity is not sustainable. Just like a diet, a fast is something that you will eventually have to curtail. If you then resort to your previous poor eating habits, you will be in for a big surprise. You will actually gain weight faster after the fast! If your body perceives that it is being starved (which it does with fasting), this triggers a protective change in metabolism that allows the muscles and tissues to conserve energy. It's as if your body says, "Wow, all the food is gone, I'd better ratchet down my needs and maximize my storage ability so I can ride this out." This means storing calories in the most efficient way, and that is fat.

During a fast, you burn glucose and fat for fuel, but once the fast is broken, your metabolism remains in a fasting mode for a period of time. So now your body, primed to save as much energy as possible, is inundated with an abundance of calories. The body then takes these excess calories, and, because of the shift in metabolism, wants to hang on to them. So the excess calories relocate to the thighs and rear end. The bottom line (pun intended) is that fasting may jump-start weight loss, but it is not a good tool for sustainable results.

> If you are one of the millions who suffer from mid-morning mood swings or a drop in energy, check out what you are eating for breakfast. Eating nothing will lead to low blood sugar by mid-morning, and eating high-sugar cereals and caffeine will cause the same symptoms. The solution is a low-sugar, protein-based breakfast.

This does not in any way discount the spiritual benefits of fasting. T. D. Jakes, well-known author and preacher, says, "Many people are discovering the pleasure of fasting and renewing the biblical advice of using a day of fasting to pray and seek direction from the Lord."[6]

IT'S NOT ABOUT DEPRIVATION

Along those lines, *how* you eat can also influence weight loss. Remember that if you approach weight loss and calorie reduction from a depravation mindset, then you are doomed to failure. Focus on all of the amazing physical and psychological benefits you will gain. Celebrate the variety of choices you do have, not what you don't have.

Train your body to respond to hunger and not the clock. Many weight loss programs correctly emphasize listening to your body and only responding when the appropriate signals are given. That means eating when your body says it needs nourishment instead of some arbitrary time or custom.

Almost all nutritionists agree that breakfast is the most important meal of the day. Our Western culture has turned this around and tends to view breakfast as the most expendable meal. Tell someone that they have to miss breakfast, and they will most likely shrug it off as an inconvenience, but tell them they must miss dinner, and you may be in for a fight. Uncommon sense dictates that breakfast (or *break* the *fast*) is critical because it fulfills two vital functions. One, it replenishes the fuel burned to maintain body functions overnight, and second, it supplies fuel to be consumed during the day. Counter this with the traditional dinner meal in which, for many persons, the most calories are consumed . . . and then we go to sleep! The logic is simple: Why not put more calories into the system when they will most likely be burned up? But instead we put the most calories in the system at a time when they will be stored. That is not to imply that you should skip dinner; just remember that it makes sense to use restraint at times of little activity. The old adage is true: Eat breakfast like a king and dinner like a pauper.

TRY SIX MEALS A DAY!

Congress has yet to pass a law mandating three meals a day. This is strictly a cultural habit and has minimal merit physiologically. Many studies have indicated that eating six small meals spaced every three to four hours is better able to keep blood sugar levels, insulin secretion, and energy levels in a more steady state. Many diabetic diets, which actually can be quite healthy for non-diabetic persons, use this approach. The key is making these *small* meals. Total calorie consumption for the day is still the most critical consideration.

Try this. Take the total calorie consumption needed for you to lose weight (from the calculations you made earlier), and then divide this total by 6. This gives you your requirement per "meal." Then plan more of the calories to be distributed in the A.M. and less in the P.M. For example, if you need 2,000 calories a day to lose weight, consider 550 for breakfast, 150 for a mid-morning snack, 550 for lunch, 200 for a mid-afternoon snack, 500 for dinner, and 50 for an evening snack. Obviously this is just an example and you would customize this based on your own needs. It will take some work initially, but you will find that it will quickly become a habit. You will also find that your energy level will be maintained throughout the day; you won't feel starved, and you won't have those bloated lulls in energy after a big meal.

A QUICK REVIEW

🏃 Step One: Determine how much you are eating currently (boo . . . hiss).

🏃 Step Two: Determine how much you need to maintain your BMR (at your goal weight) and what it would take to achieve slow, steady weight loss.

🏃 Step Three: Space these calories throughout the day, placing more in the A.M. and less in the P.M.

OR

Reduce what you are eating now by 10 percent a week until you get to the level of calories needed to maintain your BMR at your target weight.

BURN IT UP

The critical next step—step four—in the weight loss equation is to burn up more calories than you take in. Simply stated for you engineer types: Calories in − calories out = a negative number if you want to lose weight. YOU CANNOT LOSE FAT AND BE FIT WITHOUT EXERCISE! Not only does a fit person burn more calories during the exercise, but they also burn more energy at rest! What a great system! Your muscles are the greatest fat-burning machines ever created, and you develop those muscles from exercise. You exercise not so much to burn fat; you exercise to change your body's chemistry. This is such an important topic that the next chapter is solely devoted to exercise.

There you have it—a simple yet challenging plan to lose fat and keep it off. I challenge you to find any successful weight loss program that is not based on these principles: take less in, burn more off. The challenge is now yours. You are not alone, however. Millions of fellow strugglers understand your toil and frustration, so the final step in the process is to find a support network. Don't try to implement these changes alone. The success of any nutrition or exercise program is bolstered by family support. In addition, a friend, spouse, co-worker, or a formal group like Weight Watchers or Curves can provide the psychological support and accountability that breeds success. God is with you along this journey. He longs for a healthier you to fellowship with. It's not just about external appearance; it's about being whole in mind, body, and spirit.

—— FAT-PROOF POINTERS ——

Losing weight is easy: not gaining fat is hard!

There is no magic bullet, medicine, diet, or herb that will do it for you.

Take in less, burn off more.

Eat balanced, low-fat, low-sugar, high-fiber meals.

Exercise aerobically for a minimum of thirty to forty-five minutes a day (guidelines appear in next chapter).

Know your numbers: BMR and BMI.

Keep a food diary, if you dare.

Total calories matter most.

Family involvement breeds success.

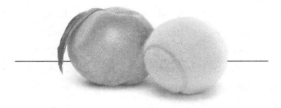

EXERCISE

SHAKE, RATTLE, **AND** ROLL

"Mom, hurry, I'm going to be late for soccer!" implored Sarah as she dashed through the kitchen.

Laurie grabbed the shin pads her daughter had forgotten and followed the pig-tailed whirlwind out to the car where they reviewed the afternoon's schedule.

"Sarah, I'll pick you up from soccer at four-thirty, then . . . hmm, it's Wednesday, so that means ballet at five-fifteen and church at six-thirty. Do you realize that I'll have spent half my day in the car today?"

"Mom, just look at it as career training. Now you can be one of those limo drivers!"

After dropping Sarah at practice, Laurie had a few minutes to grab a cup of coffee and visit with her mom, who lived nearby.

"I don't understand it," Laurie told her mom. "I'm on my feet all day, constantly on the move, yet the doctor said yesterday that I need more exercise. My first thought was, sure, I'd love to. Then I realized that I'm not sure I'd do anything, even if I had the time.

I just don't enjoy sweating, and besides, I look like the Michelin Man when I wear tights. The most organized exercise I get now is jumping to conclusions!"

"Laurie, dear, you're such a good mother, but you need to take care of yourself so you can take care of your family."

Laurie hated it when her mom was right, which she was noticing more and more. After all, this was the woman who attended her first aerobics class before it was "cool" and ran a marathon at age sixty. She was like a fine wine: more elegant with time.

"Laurie, I firmly believe that if we don't make time to exercise, we'll have to make time to be sick."

THE E WORD

At a recent seminar, I asked the audience, "If I had a pill that could make you look better, feel better, act better, lose weight, reduce your incidence of breast cancer, and was cheap, how many of you would take it?" One woman in the back began yelling like she had just been told to "Come on down!" on *The Price Is Right*.

"I want it, I want it!"

In an effort to divert her enthusiasm as she rushed toward the stage, I quickly explained, "I do have such a pill, and it's called exercise!"

> "The choice is for fitness or fatness, to exercise or not to exercise. The ultimate cure for being overweight is exercise."
>
> —Dr. George Sheehan, in *Running and Being*

She stopped dead in her tracks, sneered up at me, and said, "I want my money back!" She was suffering from the quick-fix, I-want-it-yesterday, and-I-don't-want-it-to-be-hard blues.

After regaining her composure . . . and her balance, she commented, "I'm sick of hearing about exercise. I know it is good for me—who doesn't? But it's just not something I'm going to do. If you really want to help me, give me a way to make it fun and not something I dread."

The woman was expressing the feelings shared by many people today: "I know exercise helps, but for many reasons, I just don't do it." And it was obvious from her dissatisfaction that both the medical community and the health-care industry as a whole were not meeting her needs. She is the rule rather than the exception.

For decades, doctors, experts, and fitness gurus have been preaching the far-flung benefits of regular exercise. John Dryden, an eighteenth-century poet, wrote,

> *Better to hunt in fields, for health unbought,*
> *Than fee the doctor for a nauseous draught,*
> *The wise, for cure, on exercise depend;*
> *God never made his work for man to mend.*

Nevertheless, we persist in being overweight, inactive, and unhealthy. The message is as clear as a spring day in the mountains—exercise is good for you! Yet like buckling seatbelts, *knowing what to do* doesn't always translate into *doing it*. It's like planting a seed but never watering or nourishing it, and then expecting it to flourish.

IF YOU DON'T DO, YOU DON'T GET

A brief review of the benefits of exercise is warranted because repetition is the mother of learning. The key, of course, is to apply the knowledge.

Exercise improves conditioning and fitness in healthy individuals of all ages. Translated, this means that fit individuals can do the same amount of physical exertion with a lower heart rate, breathing rate, and blood pressure than a less fit person. The practical side of this increased fitness is less risk of illness and better weight control and emotional well-being. Exercise changes body chemistry in such a way to favor keeping you fit. Exercise builds muscles, and *muscles burn fat*!

Developing and maintaining endurance is a key factor in overcoming fatigue. One of the most common problems heard in a medical office is the I'm-so-tired-of-being-tired syndrome. The three leading causes of chronic tiredness are poor nutrition, lack of exercise, and stress. This is especially prevalent in women of the reproductive age. (Do you think it has anything to do with children?) It is ironic that you may think you are too tired to exercise when it is a lack of exercise that may be a factor in your fatigue.

Exercise also enhances flexibility, or the degree to which joints and body parts can be rotated around a point. Those of you who have recently been coaxed into a game of Twister with your children understand how flexibility, or lack thereof, can provide hours of laughter for your kids and hours of pain for your joints. Stretching and flexibility are actually very important in any exercise program, and these two activities may be the keys for some in staying injury free. The famous Framingham Heart Study, which is following its third generation of research participants, has shown that losing only eleven pounds reduces the risk of osteoarthritis of the knee by 50 percent! A study published in the *American Journal of Clinical Nutrition* (March 1999) even proved that a fit overweight person had a lower incidence of heart disease that an unfit thin person!

Exercise is also well known to lower blood pressure, thwart obesity, help prevent osteoporosis, and improve your sex life with your spouse. Okay, maybe the sex-life improvement is not so well documented, but intuition should indicate it sure can't hurt it!

The benefits to the family from exercise are enormous. *The leading tool for prevention of childhood and adolescent weight problems is exercise.* Kids who are regularly active feel better, look better, act better, make better grades, and continue the habit into adulthood.

A study from the Mayo Clinic found that kids of normal weight stood and moved for an average of 368 minutes a day, compared with 282 minutes for heavy kids.

There are also many well-recognized psychological benefits of exercise. A fascinating study done in 1999 compared the effect of exercise and a frequently prescribed antidepressant on mild depression. The authors concluded, "An exercise training program may be considered an alternative to antidepressants for treatment of depression in older persons. Although antidepressants may facilitate a more rapid initial therapeutic response than exercise, after sixteen weeks of treatment exercise was equally effective in reducing depression among patients with mild depression."[1] Various studies have shown a perceived improvement in quality of life among exercisers, as well as the betterment of mood, self-confidence, and feelings of satisfaction, achievement, and self-sufficiency.

SPIRITUAL AEROBICS

My intuition is that many people have never considered exercise as a spiritual issue; however, a careful review of Scripture reveals many truths about the physical body and how vital it is to maintain. One of the most compelling and convicting passages is 1 Corinthians 6:19–20: "Don't you know that your body is the temple of the Holy Spirit, who lives in you and was given to you by God? You do not belong to yourself, for God bought you with a high price. So you must honor God with your body." These verses specifically refer to sexual immorality, but a more broad interpretation reveals its application to your physical health. The body is a temple—a holy place—set apart and meant to glorify not only its builder, but also what it houses. The Holy Spirit dwells in your body and uses this vessel as one means of accomplishing God's purpose in your life. The body functions as a conduit for the gifts of the Spirit to manifest in time and space. To honor God with your body implies not only doing what is good and healthy, but also implies refraining from that which is detrimental, both physically and spiritually.

PROZAC OR PUMPING IRON?

Frank, a good friend and business associate, was feeling down. He had encountered some financial setbacks over the previous few months and was stressed. In addition, his oldest daughter was dating a guy five years her senior, and Frank was very uncomfortable with the relationship. I noticed his sour moods at our regular breakfast get-together. Certainly he had reasons to be stressed—legitimate reasons—but Frank, being the pragmatist, was only looking for a solution. (We guys don't like to talk about our problems; we want to talk about solutions.) Frank had seen his doctor (he goes faithfully once every five years!) and the doctor had suggested Prozac. Frank was uncomfortable with this, so he asked me what I thought about antidepressant medicines. I explained that I believed there is a place for them, but as with many medicines, they are overused. I had just read a study on exercise as a tool for lifting mild depression, and I suggested Frank get back into an exercise program. He used to enjoy tennis a few years back, but had strayed when business demands took more of his time. He agreed to try exercise, knowing it wouldn't solve his dilemmas, but it might help him cope better.

A study published in the *Journal of the American Medical Association* (November 2006) shows exercise to be one of the best tools for longevity. The likelihood for a man to reach the age of eighty-five is directly related to his exercise habits in midlife.

Indeed, once Frank became committed to his morning exercise program, he was able to focus better, and he actually used the time to think through problems in a quiet setting. After two months, Frank still had some financial woes, his daughter was still dating Mr. No Good, but his ability to deal with the situations had improved. He was not depressed and seemed to have more hope for the future. The only thing that had changed was the exercise.

PONCE DE LEÓN NEEDED A TREADMILL

In addition to its other benefits, exercise is the *only* proven anti-aging tool! "If we stay active, many of the things that supposedly decline with age really don't decline," says Dr. William Simpson, aging researcher and professor of Family Medicine at the Medical University of South Carolina.[2] Dr. Terrence Kavenaugh published a study of athletes, ages thirty-five to ninety-four, competing in the 1985 World Masters games and concluded, "These men and women were more typical of the average recreational sports person rather than the elite athlete. Yet the results of their exercise habits were marked. It seems that even modest exercise can push functional aging back twenty years."[3]

There are virtually unlimited types of activities that can be used for exercise, from sitting in a chair and lifting cans of soup to joining a local health club and becoming a gym regular. So don't use the lame excuse of thinking you have to join some expensive health club to get exercise. Even if you are unemployed you can walk or run with your only expense being a well-fitting shoe. Do it regularly. Do it with the family. Make it fun.

GETTING KIDS ON THE MOVE

Actually, the necessity of involving children in exercise is a relatively new phenomenon. Until recently, kids got plenty of exercise; it was called play! Sadly, unstructured play has been uprooted by video games, computers, TV, loss of school-sponsored physical education, and kids falling into sedentary lifestyles modeled for them by their parents and others. "Childhood and physical vigor used to go together like a hand in a baseball glove," according to an article in the *University of California-Davis Health Journal*. "Most adults, no matter what racial or socioeconomic group they come from, remember childhood as a time of actively playing outdoors until darkness—and exhaustion—forced them to return home. American children today are more likely to spend much of their free time exercising little else than their fingers, as they switch channels from an easy chair or push the controls of an electronic game. Even everyday calorie-burning tasks, such as walking to school or riding a bike to visit a friend, have been replaced by car rides. Lack of exercise is a major factor in the growing problem of obesity, both for children and adults."[4]

According to the 2005 guidelines from the U.S. Department of Health and Human Services, all children two years and older should get sixty minutes of moderate to vigorous exercise on most, preferably all, days of the week. You can't rely on school physical education programs to supply this, as many have been

> Children's physical activity has a direct link to lowering their risk for later development of heart disease and diabetes, according to a study published in the British medical journal *Lancet* (July 2006). "Just making sure children play outside will double the amount of physical activity they get," says Dr. Lars Anderson.

eliminated from the curriculum of our local schools. Even reduced recess breaks are a growing trend in elementary education. According to one advocacy group, "Nearly 40 percent of the nation's

16,000 school districts have either modified, deleted, or are considering deleting recess. School districts in Atlanta, New York, Chicago, New Jersey, and Connecticut are opting to eliminate recess, even to the point of building new schools in their districts without playgrounds. Increasing demands to raise test scores and to teach more challenging curricula are among the reasons cited by school districts for eliminating recess. Schools are beginning to implement 'no recess' policies under the belief that recess wastes time that would be better spent on academics."[5]

A 1-hour-a-day school physical education program can reduce obesity in kids by 10 percent, which is significant in a world where one out of three kids born in the year 2000 will develop diabetes. A child who develops Type 2 diabetes before the age of fifteen may see a reduction of their life expectancy of twenty-seven years![6] Our kids may be smarter, but they won't live long enough to prove it!

This really is a no-brainer, except for the politicians, ivory tower academicians, and attorneys who oppose physical education programs because of budget cuts or liability concerns. If your community has eliminated physical education from the school day,

> Researchers from Cornell University recently reported that in a typical high school gym class—where there are a few jumping jacks before a game of softball—students were active for just sixteen minutes. The rest of gym time was spent being sedentary.

I encourage you to become a thorn in the side of the school board. Armed with supporting data, you can present a cogent argument for the necessity of children being active at some time during the school day (and I don't mean under the football stands!).

The following table lists guidelines published by one national organization as the minimal daily activity levels for children. These are simple guidelines that can be followed with relative ease; however, it is shocking how many of our kids don't achieve even these minimal standards. It takes two things: time and commitment. Remember, you are all about family, and that certainly applies to exercise. Shift your thinking from "me" to "us." Without a family commitment to exercise, fat-proofing falls flat. Think about a trip to a local park. You can easily spend an hour walking, hiking, throwing a ball, shooting baskets, riding bikes, or just letting the kids play while you walk. Instead of dropping the kids at soccer and leaving, walk around the field or track for an hour during the practice. When at home, let the kids play without TV and other distractions.

EXERCISE RECOMMENDATIONS FOR CHILDREN

Age	Minimum Daily Activity	Comments
Infant	No specific requirements	physical activity should encourage motor development
Toddler	1 ½ hours	30 minutes planned physical activity **AND** 60 minutes unstructured physical activity (free play)
Preschooler	2 hours	60 minutes planned physical activity **AND** 60 minutes unstructured physical activity (free play)
School age	1 hour or more	Break up into bouts of 15 minutes or more

These guidelines represent minimum *recommendations. You and your child can and should do more.*

Source: National Association for Sport and Physical Education (NASPE)

There are even exercise videos for adults and kids that you can do together, and they can be quite a workout! One group of new mothers has designed a video workout done in the home with their newborns as part of the activity. Let your imagination go.

YOU WANT ME TO DO WHAT?!

Teenagers raise the bar when it comes to being motivated to exercise. For some, exercise is an integral part of their day if they are actively involved in organized sports. For others, especially the average teen who spends almost six hours a day in sedentary activities (TV, computer, video games, studies, etc.), exercise is as welcome as zits before the prom.

It is important to remember the teenage years are times of great discovery and disjunction. They are realizing that they are unique individuals and have an almost desperate desire to assert their independence. It is a grand idea to let teens have some control over their exercise choices. Don't make the mistake of pigeonholing a teen into a specific activity because of a certain body build or competitive nature. For example, not all tall kids like basketball, and not all big kids are born football linemen. Let teens find their niche. The key is not what they are doing, but that they are doing something.

Tips for Teens—from Teens

- ⚹ If you are watching TV, exercise also (treadmills, jump rope, etc.).
- ⚹ Take the stairs instead of the elevator.
- ⚹ Get a friend to be your exercise partner.
- ⚹ Participate in after-school sports.
- ⚹ Do seasonal activites like raking leaves or shoveling snow.
- ⚹ Try an exercise video—they can be loads of fun.
- ⚹ Take your dog (or neighbor's dog) for a long walk.
- ⚹ Dance every dance at parties.
- ⚹ Help in household chores— vacuuming can be a workout!
- ⚹ Have fun in whatever you do.

Source: *teenhealthfx.com*, 2006

Teens need to have ownership of their experience, and that often means letting them select the activity. Your role is to cajole them (they may call it nagging) into picking something that they can enjoy. However, to keep them motivated long-term, it has to be fun. This is a critical point as friends have a tremendous influence on a teen's willingness to participate. Be very supportive of group activities like soccer, running, tennis, dance, and cheerleading, which involve your child's friends. Be proactive and suggest that your teen ask friends to do things with him or her and then facilitate getting it done. If you can make exercise a habit in the teen years, there is a greater chance this healthy lifestyle will continue into adulthood. Be flexible in accommodating schedules for exercise. Take them to the gym with you! The parent-chauffeur syndrome is tough at times, but the payoffs are immense if you are carting them to activities that promote fitness. Make sure they have the needed safety equipment and access to facilities that support their interest. My thirteen-year-old daughter recently expressed an interest in kickboxing. Now, this is not exactly the sport I would have chosen for her, but if she can practice it in a safe environment, I find it hypocritical for me not to support her interest.

MOTIVATING THE WHOLE FAMILY

For adults—and kids—there are two things that will successfully motivate people to change behaviors. One is achieving pleasure, and the other is avoiding pain. It will become clear that the pleasure obtained from a regular exercise program will be immense. Studies indicate, though, that the avoidance of pain is an even more motivating force. You will generally go to greater lengths to avoid pain than to gain pleasure. Write down all the painful things that will happen if you don't exercise. Personalize it and make it apply to your situation. Now make a list of all the benefits of exercise. You know most of those also: feel good, look good, live longer and happier, achieve goals, increased self-esteem, and on and on. Then do the same for the family. Put these lists in an area where everyone will see them *daily*. If you have been honest with yourself, I guarantee this reminder will be effective. Just as food should be enjoyed in moderation, so exercise must be an integral part of a varied and joyful lifestyle.

LOOK BETTER, FEEL BETTER, ACT BETTER

Joe Stamper ran on the cross-country team in high school, but after four years of typical college bad habits—fast food, late-night munching, and drinking—he graduated weighing more than two hundred pounds. Those ways continued for the next several years as he climbed the corporate ladder. When his younger brother got married right before his fortieth birthday, Stamper realized he would see many old friends and family again, and he was appalled that he now weighed 265 pounds. He realized things had gotten out of hand.

First he eliminated soda, beer, and fried foods from his diet—a painful but necessary step. He began eating breakfast again—something he had abandoned years ago—but this time with fruit and cereals instead of fast food, and he kept track of the calories he was consuming. He looked at his transition as more of a permanent change in the way he lived rather than a diet.

Most important, Joe returned to his high school sport. He decided to take up running once again. On his first outing, he ran about a quarter mile from his apartment, got winded, and had to stop and walk back home. He wasn't discouraged, though. He persisted and within four months he was regularly running four miles five days a week. In less than a year, Joe had lost nearly seventy pounds and was logging twenty to twenty-five miles a week. Now, five years later, he has maintained his regimen and feels and looks better than he did in his twenties, testimony to the dramatic life changes brought on by exercise.

JUST DO IT

The secret to exercising regularly is responsibility. We shy away from responsibility in this country. Accountability has been replaced by blame, yet this is really nothing new. Zig Ziglar is fond of telling the story about how Adam, the original artful dodger, was the first in a long line of persons to deflect the blame. When God found him in the garden and asked him about eating the apple, Adam uttered the phrase that has echoed throughout the ages: "God, let me tell you about that woman!" And when Eve was questioned, she promptly replied, "God, let me tell you about that snake!" Of course, the snake didn't have a leg to stand on!

God has given us control over the decisions affecting our bodies, and much of the health or dis-ease we encounter is the result of those choices. Never forget that God is a God who heals: "For I am the Lord who heals you," (Exodus 15:26). Can exercise be a tool for wellness? Absolutely! Can exercise be a tool for emotional well-being? Unquestionably! Can exercise be a tool for healing and reversing disease? Most assuredly! Is exercise one of the keys to fat-proofing the family? Without a doubt! God provides the tools, yet it is our responsibility to take up those tools and use them to harvest the fruits of wellness. Exercise can be a form of worship—a sacred, reverent activity meant to bring us into the presence of God. Exercise can be a way to honor and glorify the Creator by actively caring for the creation. Some of you may feel branding exercise as a means of worship is a bit of a stretch; however, worship is anything that expresses sincere gratitude and praise.

For me, running is a time of prayer. After all, prayer is communication with God, and there are times when the solitude of an early morning run brings me into a place of awe at the majesty of the One who created it all. Thus, running becomes a time of worship. There is something reverent in the constant cadence, the pattern of repetition that pervades the activity. It can be a time of quiet reflection and contemplation.

MANY FORMS

Through the ages, forms of dance—very vigorous exercise, no doubt—have been used as expressions of praise and prayer. Don't fall into the misperception that exercise is only exercise if it occurs in a smelly gym or aerobics room. This is especially important when thinking about the family. You don't have to join a gym or the YMCA to provide a place for family exercise. Use your imagination. Walking to the store or taking the stairs instead of the escalator at the mall will not only provide a brief workout, but also model healthy behavior for your children. Shift your perspective and begin to view exercise as not only a tool for creating a vibrant healthy body, but also as a means for connecting with God. Fitness is a form of praise and a joyous celebration of the Creator's masterpiece . . . you!

There are many others who share this idea of "prayerful activity." Linus Mundy founded a movement called Prayer Walking in 1985. This is a group that is committed to both physical and spiritual health by combining exercise and contemplative prayer. "Action and contemplation have always been an American characteristic," Mundy says. "By praying and walking at the same

> **Did You Know?**
> There are dozens of youth running programs across the United States that focus on participation, not necessarily competition. Some of these include Girls on the Run, Marathon Kids, the New York Road Runners Foundation, and Kids Sports Stars.

time, you really can get both spiritual and physical exercise."[7] Prayer walkers map out a route through their town, and as they are power walking they say prayers for those in the houses they pass. Mundy maintains it has literally changed communities by both promoting fitness and raising spiritual awareness.

EXCUSE ABUSE

I am constantly amazed and amused at the cunning involved in contriving reasons not to exercise. Often the effort and energy expended in rationalizing ways to avoid exercise could, if channeled more appropriately, propel you to new heights of fitness. One middle-aged man claimed, "If God had meant me to touch my toes, he would have put them closer to my knees!" You owe it to your family to disavow your excuses—and theirs—and adopt an active lifestyle today.

The vignette at the beginning of this chapter illustrates one of the most common objections to exercise. As Laurie was struggling to be everything to everyone, she was avoiding taking care of herself. As she remarked, "I just don't have the time to exercise!" What she is actually saying is, "I don't make the time to exercise." We all have the same twenty-four hours in a day, the same seven days in a week.

Imagine coming home from a long day at work. You are legitimately tired and your wife proudly announces, "Tonight is when we clean out the attic!" The whining begins immediately: "I'm so tired, and I had a busy day at work. Please, I just want to sit down." About that time the phone rings and your buddy says, "Hey, Bill, I just got a tee time, and if we hurry we can get nine in before dark." You jump up like a jack-in-the-box and exclaim, "You bet! I'll be right over!" Somehow the work fatigue instantly evaporated. Exercise is simply not a priority for most people.

The problem is not the time; it is how we choose to spend it. Many people live with the misperception that you need a one- or two-hour chunk of time to get an effective workout. This is indeed a myth, and it is scientifically proven that a much smaller block of time spent in exercise can benefit the entire family. Several recently published studies report that three ten-minute exercise sessions in a day can provide health benefits similar to a single thirty-minute session. No longer will an excuse like "Where can I possibly find the time?" be valid. Get up earlier, walk on your lunch break, take the stairs, turn off the TV. It is truly a choice.

Granted, maximal fat-burning and cardiovascular benefits are achieved with more sustained activity; however, at least some positive results can be realized with an abbreviated schedule. In fact, many who start an exercise program are better off following this pattern initially as it can be more flexible and more likely to promote consistency. It is not nearly as daunting to face a ten-minute exercise segment as it is a forty-five-minute sweat session. Like any other practice, the key is consistency. If you will exercise with your kids for fifteen-minute intervals three times a day, you will see results. Given the MTV attention span of many teens today, this approach may be your best bet for success.

Another common excuse, especially among older parents, is, "But Doc, I'm fifty and have never exercised. What good will it do me now?" The answer is simple—a great deal! You are never too old to exercise. Several studies have documented that even a ten-pound weight loss in older folks can reduce their long-term risk of medical problems. The only limiting factor is the muscle between your ears! If your doctor says you can exercise—and I would question him or her if they said otherwise—there is much to be gained from an exercise regimen tailored to your needs and abilities. Now, if you are a charter member of the couch-potato club, don't walk out the door tomorrow and run two miles. Get the proper advice from your doctor about *what you can do* (focus on that instead of what you can't do), and start slowly. In this instance, being a turtle is much more advantageous than being a rabbit. But the message is, do it! Get a good checkup, pick something you like doing, grab the kids, and for your sake, go for it!

> **Did You Know?**
> Your body burns about 50 calories a day to maintain each pound of muscle, but it only burns about 2 calories a day to maintain each pound of fat.

FANNY BLASTERS

Yet another frequent excuse for not exercising is that the equipment is too confusing or expensive. This myth has been ingrained in our consciousness, thanks to the ever-present, generally annoying infomercial. At any given moment, twenty-four hours a day, somewhere, you can view an ad for Tummy Trainers or Fanny Blasters endorsed by a soap opera celebrity who lost sixty pounds and four inches in two weeks! (Personally, I would check with her plastic surgeon!) The reality is that there is no magic piece of equipment that will produce miraculous results (see chapter 9 on scams). Certainly some devices may aid in specific exercises, but it is a myth to think that any one device is a requirement for success. People have been exercising efficiently and effectively for years without access to Thigh Beaters and Ab-O-Matics. The only equipment needed to get started is a well-fitting pair of sneakers. And no, you don't need the $250 super-air-aerobic-lighter-than-a-feather-I-can-run-faster-and-jump-higher-streaker sneaker. Don't let equipment envy thwart your efforts.

START SMALL, PLAN BIG

In 1997, at age thirty-nine, I ran my first marathon. It was 26.2 miles of joy, pain, frustration, pride, fatigue, and elation. When I began to train for this event, the longest distance I had ever run at one time was about six miles. A wise and experienced runner took me aside and gave me a piece of advice that proved to be essential in my training for and finishing the race. He said to break it down into manageable components, and the task becomes less intimidating. I didn't know if I could run twenty-six miles, but I did know I could run six. The training was a slow process of gradual improvement. Every other weekend I would run a bit farther than the previous run. The philosophy of starting small, setting a reachable goal, and building on that foundation is the key to developing any exercise program.

It doesn't matter if you are training for a marathon or starting to walk around the block. Begin with small steps. Set yourself up for success. Let each small movement in the direction of your goal be a reason to celebrate, no matter how small. Make it a priority and start today. We all know the path to hell is paved with good intentions. The path to health is paved with definite actions. If you have never exercised before, or if you have started and stopped more times than you can remember, now is the time to risk changing your life and health forever. This is a critical concept to teach your children. Gradual improvement will serve them well in many things, not just exercise.

My daughter is in the midst of studying for exams as I write this. Last night she was overwhelmed with the enormity of material she had to review. I could see the look of desperation and frustration in her eyes. We sat down this morning and designed a simple schedule for reviewing small bits at a time, eventually completing the whole task. It was still the same amount of material, but it was now perceived as manageable. It is a little trick our brain plays on itself. Have an eternal outlook on life, but manage it in daily chunks. Rich Mullins, a gifted singer and songwriter, once sang, "Live like you'll die tomorrow; die knowing you'll live forever." As Christians, we have the assurance of that coming true. Start small and plan big.

> "Small, gradual changes are easiest to follow and incorporate into your daily life. And small changes can make a big difference over time. Pick a few small changes that seem doable, for example, turning off the TV during dinner, switching from carbonated drinks to milk or water, or taking a walk after dinner once a week."
>
> Source: *www.MayoClinic.com*

WHERE TO START

If you are new to the realm of fitness, I challenge you to initially commit to ten minutes of exercise a day for a week, then work toward ten minutes twice a day for a week. Start by walking at a comfortable pace, and steadily progress to a brisk walk. Complete the third week by increasing both the time and intensity. Once you have a foundation, continue the walking, but begin to incorporate other activities described at the end of this chapter. Eventually build to forty-five minutes of brisk walking daily.

If you are having trouble finding the time, remember that each of the thirty-minute routines can be broken into segments to allow you to build to the desired duration. Be creative based on your current life situation. For example, Curt Conrad, a Cincinnati personal trainer, noticed that new moms he worked with were having problems arranging their schedules to exercise. He saw a need and came up with a program called StrollerFit in which he puts moms and their babies (in strollers) through an intense one-hour workout. The thrice-weekly regimen not only provides a great workout, but also gives the moms a chance to socialize.

On the way to family-night supper at church, Debbie, a thirty-something wife of our good friend Stan, remarked, "I would love to sign up for the new aerobics class at the gym, but I wouldn't be caught dead in those outfits. I break out in hives just thinking about spandex!" Debbie is not alone. Many women shy away from being seen in public in less than flattering outerwear, especially at the local gyms, where hard bodies and skimpy thongs are seen as admission criteria. To some, this excuse may sound trivial, but I have learned that this is a major barrier for many women.

Let me propose a couple of practical solutions. For women, consider joining a women-only health club like Curves. More and more are springing up around the country, and their success is testimony to the fact that women want to exercise in a setting where they can be comfortable and encouraged. There are also family-friendly health clubs that encourage family participation and have activities that are age specific. Remember, you don't need a club membership or spandex tights to walk in your neighborhood with the kids. Just going to a local park at times allows you the anonymity you need. Many churches are embracing health ministries and incorporating exercise programs into their schedules. A large church in our town recently completed a renovation that included a workout room that caters to families. It has become a critical part of their health ministry and a great tool for evangelism.

If the idea of being in public in tights or even a sweat suit still causes you chest pain, then begin your program in the safety and privacy of your own home. Here is where a few of the machines may be useful. A good quality, second-hand treadmill or stationary bicycle can convert a room into an instant workout center. The newspaper is full of ads for these items at reasonable rates, since most are being sold by people who bought them and then never unpacked the crates! If all else fails, just get out in the yard or walk around the block.

MORE IS OFTEN BETTER

The ideal approach is consistent, sustained aerobic activity. This type of exercise burns fat and literally changes your body chemistry. If you are already at that level, your challenge is to make small, incremental increases in either the length or intensity of your exercise. Remember, even if you are on the right path, you have to keep moving or you may get run over! A great way to realize additional improvement is either to change the routine, cross train, or set a new, specific goal. As a runner, I have found that committing to run a specific race provides an automatic goal to fuel my motivation. If I discover boredom or lack of motivation creeping into my workouts, I either change to a different activity for a while (stationary bike, ski machine, swimming, etc.), or I take a break. Be careful to set time limits on when to restart, because it is very easy to procrastinate if you haven't made that commitment. Tell your family or a friend about your plans and have them hold you accountable. Better yet, join a group (there are plenty) that exercises regularly for mutual support and accountability. Good social support is a definite predictor of success in weight loss programs, according to the National Weight Control Registry.

The greatest accountability group for exercise is the family, especially if you have teenagers! They love to hold Mom and Dad's feet to the fire (or pavement). Have a family meeting and outline your

> Iris June Vinegar started out an unlikely role model for runners. When she began running at age fifty-three, she was overweight, had high cholesterol, and hadn't exercised in years. Through persistence, great genetics, and a desire to not let age rob her of a single minute, the eighty-year-old has completed seven marathons in the last seven years.
>
> —Samantha Smith, in the *Raleigh News & Observer*

exercise plan. This is a great time to enlist their participation. As I said before, it is important for teens to have some ownership in these activities, as that will fuel their consistency. With younger children you can play the benevolent dictator as you encourage them to come along. It may be that you initially have to set the pace and begin solo, but the goal is to have the entire family participate. Most of the activities listed at the end of the chapter can be done together.

Fueling the Calorie Burn

How many calories are expended during common physical activities? The following numbers were calculated for a 154-pound person. Amounts will be higher if you weigh more than 154 pounds, and lower if you weigh less.

Moderate

Hiking	370 calories/hour
Gardening	330/h
Dancing	330/h
Golf (walking, carrying clubs)	330/h
Bicycling (<10 mph)	290/h
Walking (3.5 mph)	280/h
Weight training	220/h
Swimming (crawl, 20 yd/min)	288/h
Ballroom dancing	210/h
Canoeing (2.5 mph)	174/h
Recreational volleyball	264/h

Vigorous

Walking (4.5 mph)	460 calories/hour
Running (5 mph)	590/h
Running (6 mph)	654/h
Bicycling (>10 mph)	590/h
Aerobics	480/h
Weight training	440/h
Circuit weight training	756/h
Ice-skating (9 mph)	384/h
Swimming (crawl, 45 yd/min)	522/h
Cross-country skiing	690/h
Basketball	440/h
Tennis (recreational singles)	450/h

Source: *The Female Patient*, September 2006

Note: These numbers apply to both women and men.

Studies indicate it takes about a month of doing any activity regularly to instill it as a habit. Your goal should be initially to convince the family to give a regular exercise program a month. If they are committed and you are persistent, magic will happen. Each one of you will feel better physically and emotionally, and the family cohesiveness will improve. Make it easy and fun by keeping things light. You are not training for the Olympics! Some parents have a tendency to turn a family exercise outing into a boot camp. If that happens, prepare for a mutiny. Also, don't think that everything has to be structured. You can get caught up in being too regimented. Just because you want to spend an hour exercising doesn't mean you have to be playing a specific game or even the same game for that hour.

Children have an innate ability to make fun happen. Let them take the lead at times. If they don't want to play basketball, encourage them to walk or jump rope—and do it with them! There are many adults who would benefit greatly from a game of kick the can or capture the flag. Also keep in mind that simply having your child in an organized sport doesn't free you from the responsibility of keeping him or her active. On some teams, especially if your child is not a star, he or she may spend more time standing around or on the bench than actually moving.

If you love to exercise, remember that the benefits toward fitness are linear—up to a point. In other words, if you increase the duration or intensity of exercise, you will increase your fitness level.

GET PERSONAL

An exercise regimen must be individualized. Focus on what you can do, not what restrictions you have. Too many times people begin by asking, "What are the things I shouldn't be doing?" But what you should be asking is, "What *can* I do?"

Bob Hope once said that middle age is when your age starts to show around your middle! If that is the case, then exercise is your best middle-age makeover. For an exercise regimen to be maintained, it must be convenient, reasonably fun, and results-oriented. Most folks have a difficult time continuing anything that doesn't produce some positive reinforcement. This is why it is so important to look at the individual goals of each family member and set very specific parameters to measure success. It may be a certain weight or an ability to go a certain distance. Individualize your goals and keep them handy to provide motivation and success monitoring. Have family goals as well as individual goals, and write them down. Psychologists have long known that written goals are much more motivating than just a mental picture. Post them on the refrigerator for all to see. Remember, goals must be specific, timed, realistic, and personalized. For example: "I want to walk three miles a day in forty minutes by four months of starting a walking program."

First Things First

There are some important caveats to beginning an exercise program. Always have a good physical exam before instituting any regimen. Now, don't let this dissuade you from starting immediately! If your exam is not scheduled for six months, at least begin a walking program now. I know of very few people, regardless of their medical condition, who can't walk for ten to thirty minutes. Once you understand your *lack* of limitations, learning what to do is simple. Most health clubs will have people who will assist you in correctly using machines and weights if you choose that route.

If you know how to walk, you can begin an exercise program. If you can take your pulse, you can monitor the intensity of the exercise and check your progress. It is that simple. And if you have no pulse, then exercise won't help you much anyway!

HARD AND EASY

Two final concepts that are critical to fat-burning fitness and visible results are intensity and rest. The secret to efficient fitness is making the exercise *aerobic* and *sustained*. Aerobic means with oxygen, and this element is absolutely essential in the metabolism of fat. Your level of fitness is literally how well your muscles burn oxygen. A simple way of determining whether the exercise is aerobic is to measure your pulse while exercising and, if it is above 110, you are doing something right. However, and this is just as important, you should always be able to carry on a conversation while you are exercising. If you are too out of breath to do this, you are exercising anaerobically, which will not get rid of fat. You need to slow down.

The second component to fat-burning aerobic exercise is sustained activity. Studies show that to attain maximal fat-burning, you must exercise aerobically for a minimum of twenty minutes. There are many things you can do that will build strength, protect bones, and contribute to overall health other than aerobic exercise. Weight lifting is rarely an aerobic exercise, but it can be very beneficial to you in all seasons of life, especially when dealing with osteoporosis prevention. Yoga, stretching, and Pilates are great exercises, but they are rarely aerobic.

Rest is an essential component of any exercise program. It is actually during the rest periods that muscle is built and repaired. A fit person's body is burning more fat than a non-fit person's, even at rest! As you build your lean body mass (muscle), you increase the number of fat calories required to maintain that muscle. So even when you are sleeping, a fit person's body is burning more fuel to maintain and repair the often-used muscles. Recovery time from intense exercise may increase with age, so be sensitive to your body's needs. Slow down and allow for healing if your body tells you to.

LET'S GET MOVING!

For practical reasons, I have divided the exercise programs into logical age groupings:

🚶 Children (young at heart)

🚶 13–25 years old (still young and loving it)

🚶 26–40 years old (hey, I'm almost forty!)

🚶 41–50 years old (hey, I'm almost fifty!)

🚶 51 years and older (hey, I'm not going downhill; I'm picking up speed!)

Because each age group has specific goals and needs, each program is designed to meet the challenges of that era. Whenever you group such knowingly diverse individuals into categories, certain assumptions are made. Even so, experienced coaches know that the needs of the individual are similar enough that the workout regimens have validity. You will develop your own goals; therefore, every program needs to be molded to your needs while still incorporating the family dynamics. These suggested workouts serve as a template upon which an individualized program can be constructed. However, many people are satisfied to follow them specifically, with excellent results. Remember, you must include family members in your exercise regimen. Modeling is the best teacher.

CHILDREN

Refer back to the table on page 157 that outlines minimum activity levels for children. A quick summary shows that kids should get sixty minutes of planned physical activity AND sixty minutes of unstructured physical activity (free play) daily. Understand these are minimum requirements. Also keep in mind that many youngsters are not getting any recess or physical education at school. If your kids are, ask what they are doing and how long they spend in the activities. As I mentioned before, if physical education has gone by the wayside in your school district, fight for its reinstatement.

Kids at this age don't need a formal exercise plan. They get plenty of exercise if they are allowed to play. That involves two things on your part: providing the opportunity and the incentive. Make sure they have a safe environment to run around and play, whether that is the backyard or the local park, and make sure they have access to it. This may involve some sacrifice and time on your part, but you can do it out of love and the knowledge that you are creating a legacy of health.

Next, you must create the incentive to play because there are so many distractions in today's world. Turn off the TV, computer, video games, and iPods and turn on the hula hoops, ice skates, Rollerblades, and basketballs. It is the parent's responsibility to push, prod, and poke the child to be active, as this may not be their natural tendency. The secret weapon is *your* participation, especially if there are no peers around to play with. Get out with them and have some fun yourself. There is nothing like kicking a ball to work off a little frustration!

13–25 YEARS OLD

Many lifelong habits are established in this important time in a person's life. Studies indicate that men and women who are fit and active at these ages tend to continue to exercise throughout their life. Exercise becomes a habit that is hard to break! If you are long past this era, don't fret—it is never too late to start.

Teens are physically able to do many of the structured activities that adults master, so this is a great opportunity to work together, especially if your teen shows an interest in a particular sport. One of my daughters has become interested in basketball, and some of our most meaningful times together are on our driveway as she takes it to her old dad. There was a great scene in the remake of the movie *Father of the Bride* where Steve Martin's character is struggling with how to deal with his older daughter getting married. She is outside one evening shooting baskets alone, and he joins her for a game of one-on-one. It stirs fond memories of times past and allows them to feel the strength of the bond they have developed, and this then provides the opening to see eye-to-eye. This reconciliation was all possible because of the time spent in earlier years creating treasured memories shooting hoops.

Men and women of this age are generally more focused on body image rather than long-term health consequences. Therefore, these routines are geared more toward fat-burning and strength training. Even though the primary focus is on external appearance, internally the body is reaping the benefits and laying the foundation for long-term health.

An additional benefit for women from regular exercise in this age group is a major reduction of PMS (premenstrual syndrome) symptoms. Actually, this is an indirect benefit for men also! PMS is a real, medically recognized problem that is intimately linked to a woman's cycle. It is characterized by either physical or emotional symptoms (or often both) that revolve around the luteal phase, or second half, of the cycle. Medical science is rapidly answering questions surrounding the cause and treatment of PMS, but all researchers agree that exercise is a cornerstone of therapy. Regular exercise releases various hormones, such as the endorphins, that have a profound effect on the brain, primarily in the areas that control moods and emotions. Exercise is also known to help alleviate mild depression, largely through the same mechanism. The early years of the reproductive cycle are often when the first signs of menstrual-related emotional and physical changes first appear. Pursuing a consistent fitness lifestyle can reduce these changes.

If you are unsure of the terminology on some of the following exercises, consult one of the books in the Additional Resources section, or better yet, work with a friend or family member who can teach you the proper form and intensity. Check the appendix for some simple instructions on weight-lifting exercises.

Monday:	Brisk walk for 30 minutes at 70 percent of your maximal heart rate (220 − your age = maximal heart rate)
Tuesday:	Weight training. Start with light weights (5 lbs) you can find at any sports store and gradually progress to higher weights. Do 8 to 12 repetitions of each exercise.

	Upper Body Exercises:
	    Arm curls Shoulder presses
	    Lateral raises Abdominal crunches
	    Bench presses

Wednesday:	30 minutes to an hour of aerobic activity (walking, stationary bicycle, running, step class, etc.) for 30 minutes to an hour.

Thursday:	Lower Body Exercises:
	    Lunges Calve raises
	    Squats Abdominal crunches
	Do 8 to 12 repetitions of each exercise.

Friday:	30 minutes to an hour of aerobic activity
Saturday:	30 minutes of aerobic activity followed by 15 minutes of stretching
Sunday:	Rest

Keep in mind that a thirty- to sixty-minute aerobic activity can be divided into fifteen-minute chunks if your schedule demands. You will get maximum benefit from continuous activity, however.

26–40 YEARS OLD

During these years many couples are considering starting or adding to their family. Some couples are concerned about the effect of exercise on their fertility. There are no good studies to date that support the idea that fit individuals have a different fertility rate than their inactive counterparts. The exception is the woman who exercises to the degree that her periods cease. Even in these individuals ovulation can occur, which in turn could lead to pregnancy. This degree of exercise intensity is relatively rare and is most commonly seen in competitive athletes. In general, exercise has little impact, positive or negative, on pregnancy rates. If you are an avid exerciser and are having trouble getting pregnant, you may consider decreasing the intensity or duration of your activity, especially if you tend to have irregular menstrual cycles.

Exercise during pregnancy is also an important consideration of this age group. If you are fit prior to pregnancy, you can continue to exercise during your pregnancy.

"In the absence of either medical or obstetrical complications, pregnant women can continue to exercise and derive related benefits," according to the American College of Obstetricians and Gynecologists. "Women who have achieved fitness prior to pregnancy should be able to safely maintain that level of fitness throughout the pregnancy and the post-partum period."[8]

SAMPLE EXERCISE PROGRAM FOR PREGNANCY

This is a simple regimen for women who didn't exercise much prior to getting pregnant. It is a good starting place for the uninitiated. Always check with your doctor before starting any exercise program.

Monday:	Brisk walking for 45 minutes
Tuesday:	Water aerobics or stationary bike for 45 minutes
Wednesday:	Brisk walking for 45 minutes
Thursday:	Weight training with light weights. Focus on upper body by doing exercises such arm curls, lateral raises, and bench presses. Avoid lunges and abdominal crunches.
Friday:	Brisk walking for 45 minutes
Saturday	Water aerobics or stationary bike for 30 to 45 minutes
Sunday	Rest

For all you folks who are not concerned about pregnancy (okay men, I realize you are feeling neglected at this point), I generally recommend following the same regimen outlined in the 13- to 25-year-old section. Again, realize these are guidelines for someone just beginning an exercise regimen. Many of you will be much more advanced than this, and in that case, keep on doing what you are doing. Work more toward incorporating your family into your activities. Experienced exercisers may need to increase either the intensity or duration to continue to see positive gains in their fitness. As you age, your caloric requirements to maintain normal body functions declines, so to keep balanced you have to burn up more if your intake is the same. That means either eating less or smarter, or exercising harder or longer (or both).

41–50 YEARS OLD

One of the greatest benefits of fitness in these years is the prevention of maladies brought on by aging.

People in this age group are only limited in what they can do by their current health status. An important caveat for this time frame is to include some weight-bearing exercises to help in osteoporosis prevention.

Monday:	Aerobic activity (aerobics, running, brisk walking, etc.) for at least 45 minutes; more is better.
Tuesday:	Weight training, focusing on the major muscle groups. Bench presses for the pectorals, arm curls for the biceps, lateral raises for the back, crunches for the abdominals, leg extensions for the quads, and squats for the rump roast. Here is where a good instructor can walk you through the exercises and make sure you are doing them correctly for maximal benefit.
Wednesday:	Aerobics for 30 to 45 minutes. (Cross-training is excellent, so if you are used to only walking or running, try changing for a while to swimming or biking or in-line skating, etc.)
Thursday:	Weight training again
Friday:	Consider some form of team sport such as volleyball, basketball, or water polo. Many groups such as the YWCA and YMCA have great team programs.
Saturday:	Aerobic activity for 30 to 45 minutes, ideally with the family
Sunday:	Rest

51 YEARS AND OLDER

This is the age that will encompass the menopause for most women and mental pause for most men. In some women this hormonal shift may trigger physical and emotional alterations that can vary from mildly annoying to life disrupting. Through all of these variations, you can find solace in exercise. Countless scientific studies have shown marked improvement in symptoms, such as hot flashes, with the introduction of a simple exercise regimen. Exercise is also critical in these years to prevent osteoporosis and heart disease. Those who are active feel better about themselves and others.

In this age group the focus is on cardiovascular health and flexibility.

Monday:	Brisk walk for at least 45 minutes
Tuesday:	Pilates, or some other form of active stretching, for at least 30 minutes
Wednesday:	Light weights for bone health (a combination of both upper and lower body exercises)
Thursday:	Aerobic activity for at least 45 minutes. (Water aerobics is especially good for those with joint problems and arthritis.)
Friday:	Stretching activity for at least 30 minutes
Saturday:	Aerobic activity for at least 45 minutes
Sunday:	Rest

Keep in mind these programs are merely suggestions and targeted to the beginner. There will be many of you that individually are able to do much more than what is described here, but I'll bet someone in the family is a beginner. All of these regimens are proven and effective, but none will work without the key ingredient . . . YOU! The road to "someday" inevitably leads to nowhere. Make exercise a priority. Make exercise a tool. Make exercise a family celebration. Make exercise a fat-proofing fuel. Make exercise worship! Now, put down the book and get moving . . . today!

—— FAT-PROOF POINTERS ——

The ultimate cure for being overweight is exercise.

Shift your thinking from "me" to "us."

Without a family commitment to exercise, fat-proofing falls flat.

A one-hour-a-day school physical education program can reduce obesity in kids by 10 percent, which is significant in a world where one out of three kids born in the year 2000 will develop diabetes.

Peers play an influential role in your child's life at this point, so create opportunities for them to be active with their friends.

Two things will successfully motivate people to change behaviors: achieving pleasure and avoiding pain.

There are many well-recognized psychological benefits of exercise.

Exercise is the only proven anti-aging tool.

The secret to exercising regularly is responsibility.

Three ten-minute exercise sessions in a day can provide health benefits similar to a single thirty-minute session.

It doesn't matter if you are training for a marathon or starting to walk around the block; begin with small steps.

The greatest accountability group for exercise is the family.

Have family goals as well as individual goals, and write them down.

The secret to efficient fitness is making the exercise aerobic and sustained.

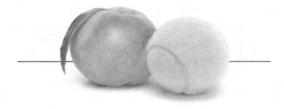

BEWARE

SNAKE OIL, **SCAMS**, AND RUBBER WRAPS

No area of health care is more fraught with misinformation, misuse, and outright fraud than the weight loss and fitness industry. To make good decisions, you must separate the wheat from the chaff. In dealing with scam diets, bogus nutritional supplements, and unhealthy practices, knowledge is power. In this chapter, I will explore fad diets (explaining why they don't work and how they can be dangerous), the myth of supplements, the dangers of prescription weight loss aids, and various other weight loss scams. You must be cognizant of these shenanigans to protect your family and your wallet.

In this age of quick fixes and McSolutions, scavenging for a shortcut to solve problems is routine. The I-want-it-and-I-want-it-yesterday mentality oozes over into health care and the weight loss industry in particular. The dollars involved are staggering. Figures from 2001 showed that Americans spent 50 billion dollars that year alone on diet products.[1] This exceeds the projections for the entire federal education, training, employment, and social services budgets by 5 to 10 billion dollars. In fact, this figure is the equivalent of the gross national product of Ireland!

"How can the diet industry keep making more and more money, year after year? Fifty billion dollars is a lot of cash!" says Tracie Johanson, a fitness expert. "The answer to that question is simple: repeat business. Ninety-eight percent of today's dieters gain the weight back in five years. Ninety percent of those individuals end up gaining back more than they lost originally, due to the body's panic and efforts to stabilize metabolic rates over the long term."[2]

> "Each time we go on another diet of deprivation, the weight becomes more difficult to lose, and we become even more frustrated and discouraged. Then we eat more and exercise less, causing ourselves more frustration, discouragement, depression. Soon we are in a vicious cycle."
>
> —Tom Venuto, BS, personal trainer

How do the diet promoters corral all that repeat business? The weight loss industry is a very unique enterprise in that when it fails you, you rarely blame the product. I am hard-pressed to find another business where, if the product doesn't work, we blame ourselves. The tendency is for us to believe that we failed the diet rather than the other way around. That is absurd! But that's exactly what we do when it comes to diets.

There is one thing that all the weight loss pills, potions, gadgets, and devices have in common: They are all selling hope. But it is a false hope—a hope that there is a secret to shorten the path to real results. A hope that is based on placebo effects, sham science, and misplaced trust. "Gee, wouldn't it be great if this really works! I think I'll give it a try." Think for a moment. If any one of these products actually was successful long-term, it would be on every TV station, magazine, and media outlet imaginable. That hasn't happened because such a product, program, or diet doesn't exist. True hope lies in the only proven, long-term solution that has never been maligned or discounted: nutritionally balanced eating and smart exercise.

The weight loss industry and snake oil salesmen prey not only on our naiveté but also on our guilt. We know that being unfit and overweight is unhealthy, and cognitively we want to do something about it. Weight loss purveyors are master promoters, and they design products and services that sound appealing but rarely deliver. People who succumb to the diet *du jour* and the weight loss miracle product of the week are both victims, and at times, willing accomplices. They are victims in that they are being sold a fraudulent, sometimes dangerous package of goods and services; and they are accomplices by not doing their homework and determining what is legitimate and what is bogus.

I want to be clear in that this is not an indictment of all weight loss products and services. It would be wrong to impugn all the various items and plans available. I want to say explicitly that there are some great programs that help in weight management; you just have to evaluate each on their own merits.

ASK THE TOUGH QUESTIONS

There are some general guidelines that everyone should apply when analyzing a weight loss or fitness product or service. Either you take the time to research a product, or you take the time to make the money that you threw away on a worthless endeavor.

- 𝕏 **Do you have to follow a specific meal plan that doesn't allow variation?** Some things are just not practical and will not be able to be sustained over time, especially for the whole family.

- 𝕏 **Do you have to purchase special food, drugs, or supplements?** Watch here for major costs. Many scam programs make most of their money by promoting their own brand of food items that are of equal or lesser quality. Often the prices are far greater than you would pay for something comparable in the grocery store.

- 𝕏 **Does the program include exercise or provide exercise instruction?** If it doesn't, run away; it might be the only exercise you will get with this program. Again, fitness cannot be achieved by dieting alone. There are a lot of sick, skinny people in the world!

- 𝕏 **Who supervises the program?** Is the instructor the kid from down the street who needed a summer job to pay for his cigarettes?

🏃 **Do participants talk with a doctor (preferably one with a medical degree who knows something about nutrition)?** Many programs employ doctors to sign forms and give the appearance of legitimacy. Often the client never sees a physician, yet they get a "blood panel" and "recommendations" from a doctor . . . who is trained in dermatology!

🏃 **What is the total cost of the program?** I mean *all* the costs, including special assessments or add-ons once you have paid the initial fees for blood tests, supplements, renewals, etc.

🏃 **Is there any accountability?** How much weight does an average participant lose, and how long does he or she keep the weight off? Don't accept testimonials. These are always exceptions that are never characteristic of the average Joe or Josie. Just like the info-mercials, these programs will have a disclaimer after every testimonial that the reported results are unusual and your results may vary. That is a true statement, but terribly incomplete. You are much more likely to be in the average group. Get those figures.

I guarantee that if you gather even some of this information on a program you are considering, you will be successful in determining whether it is legitimate or bogus. There is no excuse for anyone to purchase a product or sign up for a program without first assessing its viability. The resources are available; you only have to supply the time and effort. Don't rely solely on information supplied by the seller. There is an intrinsic bias in any information originally printed to persuade. Seek independent resources for honest critiques of the product or service. Search engines on the Internet provide a wealth of sources for investigating a particular product.

The fact is that there is no magic bullet, no holy grail of weight loss. Remember from kindergarten:

Amounts matter.
We need our brain in the game.
Discipline reaps rewards.
Exercise (play) is essential.
Rest is needed.
It's not about restrictions.

Variety leads to perseverance and success.
That family that plays together, stays together.
God is our Rock and Redeemer

Asking the right questions and mining reliable information will eliminate many of the programs on the market today.

SCAMwatch, an Australian consumer watchdog group, has compiled a list of things to watch for in a program, device, or product. It's likely to be a scam if it . . .

- ✗ Lacks scientific evidence or demonstrated links between the result and the effects of the program, food, supplement, gadget, or process being promoted.

- ✗ Is sold outside normal commercial distribution channels such as only through the Internet, by unqualified individuals, multi-level marketers, or mail-order advertisements.

- ✗ Claims effortless, large, or fast weight loss such as "lose 30 pounds in 30 days," "lose weight while you sleep," and "lose weight and keep it off for good."

- ✗ Claims to achieve weight loss without exercise, or without managing food or energy intake.

- ✗ Fails to recommend medical supervision, particularly for low-calorie diets.

- ✗ Claims to reduce fat or cellulite in specific areas.

- ✗ Uses emotive terms such as "miraculous exclusive breakthrough."

- ✗ Recommends the exclusive use of any type of gadget.

- ✗ Claims to be a treatment for a wide range of ailments and nutritional deficiencies.

- ✗ Promotes a particular ingredient, compound, or food as the key factor of success.

- ✗ Demands large advance payments or long-term contracts.

Source: *www.scamwatch.gov.au*

NATURAL PRODUCTS

Before you are tempted to buy the newest weight loss herb or pill, do this simple exercise: Carefully look at the advertisement or packaging, and search for the statement "works in conjunction with a reasonable diet and exercise," or "these claims have not been evaluated by the FDA and this product is not intended to treat any particular illness." You will find these statements somewhere in their ads or on their packaging because their lawyers demand it. Let's face it, *any* herb, potion, or product will work when combined with a sensible diet and exercise, but it happens to be the diet and exercise—not the gimmick—that is working! Also realize that none of the herbal or "natural" products are regulated by the FDA (U.S. Food and Drug Administration), unlike prescription medicines. That means you must depend on the goodwill of the company to stand behind its claims. And if you think most of these product manufacturers are concerned with your success rather than your dollars, you may also believe that airlines are always on time and you can't get fat from eating off other people's plates!

"CHRISTIAN" HUCKSTERS

It grieves me to acknowledge that some of the worst purveyors of misinformation and sham products for weight loss—and health in general—are in the so-called Christian marketplace. This whole phenomenon of Christian marketing has only been with us for a relatively short time. In years past, it was rare to have anything overtly labeled or identified as Christian because it actually thwarted marketing efforts. This is no longer the case. The Christian audience, largely due to new inroads into the media, is inundated by advertising campaigns. This is a huge market segment that has the demographics that appeal to everyone from authors to vitamin manufacturers.

Conservatives and Christians (and they are not necessarily the same) saw the post-modern relativism of the '60s as a total affront to their lifestyle and beliefs. They also recognized, for the good, that their religious beliefs transcended their everyday lives to encompass all aspects of their existence. Christianity was no longer something talked about and practiced only on Sundays; it became a worldview, a way of perceiving events. Likewise, the advent of TV stations, radio broadcasts, newspapers, and magazines with overtly Christian precepts and visions changed the environment where things are sold and marketed. Being labeled "Christian" has turned from a market-ing death blow to a cash cow. A whole new audience suddenly appeared for products, programs, books, and music.

Let me be very clear. I think this emerging attention to all things Christian is generally a good thing. I believe with my heart that all aspects of our lives are impacted by our particular worldview. This book itself is labeled as a Christian book (and is published by a Christian pub-lisher) because it proclaims the belief in Christ as Lord of your health as well as your heart, and rightly so. In reality there are no Christian books; there are books that speak truths with a Christian worldview.

The top five weight loss scams according to WebMD are:

* Metabolism-boosting pills based on herbal ingredients
* Fat- and carb-blocking pills
* Herbal weight loss teas
* Diet patches, jewelry, or other products worn on the body
* Body wraps or "slim suits"

When I am being critical, I am directing that criticism at those who cloak themselves in their Christianity to add legitimacy to what they are saying. It is the sham credibility of products and services that would otherwise be labeled as inferior that creates the problem. Among believers, there is a properly placed trust and understanding that lies at the heart of the community. There is no doubt that your word is your bond. The apostle Paul said, "Don't lie to each other, for you have stripped off your old evil nature and all its wicked deeds. In its place you have clothed yourselves with a brand-new nature that is continually being renewed as you learn more and more about Christ, who created this new nature within you" (Colos-sians 3:9–10).

There are some persons, products, and services in the health and wellness industry that have no data, no experience, no scientific basis, and no credibility. So they adopt the only moniker that will facilitate their legitimacy: they say they are a Christian company or a Christian product, or they advertise on Christian TV. As a physi-cian and a Christian, I am especially skeptical of these folks who hide under the auspices of being "Christian." I say all this simply to encourage you to evaluate every product or program on its merits, not a particular label. Don't fall into the fallacy of believing, "If it's promoted by Christians, for a Christian audience, it has to be good, effective, or inexpensive." It may be all of those things, but it should be able to stand on its merits. In my mind, being labeled as Christian actually holds it to a higher standard than its secular counterparts.

I have a friend who is a Christian illusionist, and he is fond of saying that the greatest praise he can give God is to be the best at what God has equipped him to be. In his case, he doesn't want to be a good Christian illusionist; he wants to be a great illusionist who is a Christian. Both his witness and his legacy depend on it. In the same way, I don't want to be an author and doctor that is any less competent than my secular colleagues or, more important, hide my incompetence behind a label. I give glory to God by being the best I can be with the gifts and graces I am given.

Indeed, there are wonderful secular and Christian companies and programs dedicated to health and wellness. I encourage you to hold both to the highest standards.

DIET OF THE MONTH CLUB

I want to address three arenas where the most grievous examples of abuse exists: fad diets, gadgets, and herbs and vitamins.

A recent Federal Trade Commission report found that more than half of the weight loss ads that ran in 2001 made at least one false or unsubstantiated claim.[3] Many made far more than one. We are inundated with advertisements and testimonials of a "breakthrough" discovery or a "miracle" food. The millionaire club has swelled its ranks with the diet gurus of the twenty-first century. Every celebrity has his or her own diet plan, and the wackier the better. And in places like Beverly Hills, M.D. now stands for "My Diet."

You have heard all the catchy names—South Beach, Atkins, Scarsdale, Beverly Hills, and so on. In fact, one search estimated that there has been over seventeen thousand diet books published! There is one thing they all have in common: slick marketing. Have you ever wondered why there are so many super diets, and why they arrive on the scene so frequently? The simple answer is DIETS

DON'T WORK! To be fair, I should clarify that by saying diets don't work long-term. A diet is something you initiate with the intention of someday (usually sooner than later) terminating. The logic is clear. If eating a particular way forced you into needing a certain diet, then going back to that style of eating after you have "finished" the diet will re-create the original problem. This inevitable pattern is known as the yo-yo effect, and it is the basis for the yearly trend of publishing the newest blockbuster diet. Statistically, marketers understand that by the time another year rolls around, most of those who jumped on the prior year's diet will have long given up and are now looking for the next great way to lose. And lose they do, in their health and pocketbooks! No other industry has the numbers of repeat customers as do the weight loss factories, and this alone creates health problems. University of Michigan health researchers report, "Those who gain and/or lose at least ten pounds in a year-long period at least five times over a lifetime may be setting themselves up for heart problems. So even if a woman in our study was now thin, getting there by yo-yo dieting was shown to have a negative affect on the blood flow to her heart."[4]

In honor of past fallen diets, here are some lesser known diets that never made it into the mainstream:

The Augusta Diet: You eat only birdies and eagles.

The Hypocrisy Diet: You eat only crow.

The New York Diet: You can eat anything you want as long as it is always in your face.

The Chicago Diet: Strictly meat, mainly bears and cubs.

The Nashville Diet: Eat anything corny, then pick and grin.

The Doctor Diet: Eat only rich food and scream when you get the bill.

The Lawyer Diet: Eat anything, then lie about it.

The Preacher Diet: Talk only about things you can't eat and back it up with Scripture and amusing anecdotes.

Because of the abundance of "named" diets, it is neither possible nor preferable to analyze and critique them individually (my lawyer agrees), and actually, it makes little sense to do so as they will likely be dust in the wind by the time this book hits bookstores. Most diets have the longevity of a beer at a ballgame and the utility of a screen door on a submarine.

With that being said, let's look at some categories of popular diets and briefly examine their claims.

LOW-CARBOHYDRATE/HIGH-PROTEIN DIETS

These types of diets cycle like locusts and hemorrhoids. They go away for a while, then resurface every few years. Examples include Atkins, Protein Power, Carbohydrate Addict, Sugar Busters, and The Zone. The reason they resurrect is not because they work, but because it takes a while for those who failed on them before to quit caring about it. Many of these diets focus on the interaction of carbohydrates, insulin, and fat. Essentially they claim that carbohydrates are converted to fat in the body by insulin, a hormone secreted by the pancreas. This is absolutely true. But you can't stop there. The carbohydrates that are broken down into sugars and converted into fat are only those in excess of what the body needs. This is a critical distinction. If you take in more than you need, or don't burn off more than you take in, the fat gets created and stored on your thighs and other unwanted areas! The converse is true also. If you take in less and burn off more, the excess fat is not made. It is about calories, regardless of the source.

The type of calories you consume does matter, but not as much as the total amount. Most people will lose weight initially on these types of diets because they are restricting their calories, not because they are restricting a particular type of food.

Another problem with this category of diets is their inability to be sustained. People just can't eat this way long-term. In addition, data is appearing that says it may not be healthy over the long haul to pump in excessive protein. We are talking about lifestyle here, so if a way of eating gives short-term results but long-term complications, is it really beneficial? In fact, recent scientific data should drive the popularity of these types of diets to the level of boils and baldness.

A 2003 review of Atkins-like "theories" in the *Journal of the American College of Nutrition* concluded: "When properly evaluated, the theories and arguments of popular low-carbohydrate diet books . . . rely on poorly controlled, non-peer-reviewed studies, anecdotes and non-science rhetoric. This review illustrates the complexity of nutrition misinformation perpetrated by some popular press diet books. A closer look at the science behind the claims made for [these books] reveals nothing more than a modern twist on an antique food fad."[5]

To date there have been four studies that looked at the long-term effect of these low-carb diets, and not a single one showed significantly more weight lost at the end of the year on these programs than on the control "low-fat" diets.[6]

An additional criticism of these low-carbohydrate/high-protein diets is the exclusion of many known healthy foods such as fruits, vegetables, and whole grains. If you refer back to the chapter on basic nutrition (chapter 4), you will find that many of these substances have long been validated by science as not only healthy but essential for fat-proofing your family.

The Zone is complex and has a substantial list of "forbidden" foods. Its biggest criticism is that the diet is simply too complex to follow.

Sugar Busters says excess sugar increases the level of insulin in the body and increases the likelihood of food being stored as fat. While this may be partially true, it is only a piece of the puzzle.

Protein Power says by keeping carbohydrate intake low and protein intake high, your body will burn fat faster and not feed it. However, scientific research shows being overweight is not a result of insulin levels being high, but that being overweight causes insulin problems.

The data does support the *short-term* (< six months) effectiveness of these types of diets, but keep close to your heart that you are not interested in a quick fix. You and your family are in it for life! A recent study of over nine thousand people done by the Centers for Disease Control found that in their sampling, only about 25 percent of people on a low-carbohydrate diet remained on the diet at one year, and only 10 percent were still eating this way at two years![7]

"EAT ONLY CARDBOARD" DIETS

What about diets that focus on the overconsumption of certain types of foods? These include programs such as the Beverly Hills and South Beach diets. These diets suffer many of the same problems as the low-carbohydrate diets, mainly unsubstantiated claims and long-term side effects. These types of programs depend largely on testimonials of satisfied users to lend credibility to their claims. Anecdotes or testimonials are as useful as thermal underwear in the desert! If the only evidence of the effectiveness of a diet is how well Aunt Gertrude did while on it, save your money and buy Aunt Gertrude a Twinkie, because chances are that is what she is eating now that she is off the diet. Again, most of these diets will help you lose weight in the short term, not because of any special formula, but because they restrict calories. They are not sustainable nor are their losses. Any diet that restricts healthy choices and bestows some magical properties to one type of food is nutritionally unsound.

The South Beach Diet was created for the purpose of lowering cholesterol for heart patients and those with diabetes. Such a diet is simply going to lower caloric intake for those who follow it, hence weight loss occurs.

I also place programs that require you to purchase food from a particular source in this category. What a setup for failure! Not only are the items often expensive, but they are totally impractical for the family. Imagine telling your teen that tonight, and every night, she is going to have "Healthy Eating boil-in-a-bag Tofu." I suspect she would run away, as she should.

How to Identify a Healthy Eating Program

- ✗ Sound independent research supports the claims (not just testimonials from the company).
- ✗ A well-balanced diet that is not too restrictive or difficult to follow. (God has provided an abundance; variety is good.)
- ✗ Exercise is an important part of the plan, and not just mentioned briefly in passing. (Just do it!)
- ✗ The plan makes no magical claims of easy weight loss. However, the strategies the program promotes are the most time-tested ones that lead to permanent losses and lifelong changes. (Eating nutritionally and exercising can be challenging, but so is heart disease and diabetes.)
- ✗ The plans are safe to follow. (You won't grow a third arm and turn yellow.)

Source: *www.dietchannel.com* (2006), commentary my own

SHOCKING DEVICES

Late last week I was hibernating in my on-call cubicle (a small room in the hospital that resembles a prison cell), waiting for a baby to be born, and I flicked on the TV. (I needed to be numbed at this point.) I encountered an infomercial for a device that "shocks" the muscles, causing them to contract, and, according to the announcer, gives you washboard abdominals. The swimsuit model looked like she was having a localized seizure with her tummy jumping around with each "shock." I thought to myself, *Is this what it has come to? Are we so brain-dead as a society that this type of device sells thousands of units?*

The commercial reminded me of an incident when I was an intern. One of the patients we had just operated on was experiencing intense pain around her incision. One attending physician suggested we use a TENS unit on her belly to lesson the pain. A TENS unit is an electrical stimulator that sends a small current through the skin that blocks some of the pain response. It is a scientifically valid tool for reducing pain, and the electric current can be regulated by a dial, much as you would turn up or down the volume on a radio. I was unfamiliar with the device (come on, I was just an intern), so the next morning, when I was making my rounds and the patient commented that the device didn't seem to be working—that she was still in a great deal of pain—I surmised that I simply needed to dial up the device to give a better effect. This was my first mistake. I reached over and cranked up the dial, effectively sending triple the volts through her body and watched in horror as she lifted a good three feet off the bed! It was like I had stuck her with a cattle prod! When I was able to calm her down, she politely suggested that it was time for me to see other patients and leave her to recover. Being totally rattled (and completely humiliated), I obliged and continued my rounds. I did neglect to mention this event to the patient's attending physician, who was going to see her a bit later in the day. This was my second mistake. When he saw her, she mercifully didn't comment on our encounter and calmly told him that she didn't think the device was working well. So he proceeded to reach over and crank up the device himself. After she was peeled off the ceiling, they both agreed that maybe morphine was a better choice. So you can understand why I am a bit skeptical of such electrical devices.

In all fairness, the "abdominalizer-O-matic" does have much lower settings, and to my knowledge has not electrocuted anyone yet, but the fact remains that neither has it helped many folks. In fact, the FDA has issued the following statements regarding these and similar devices:

> *Electrical muscle stimulators are considered medical devices under the Federal Food, Drug, and Cosmetic Act. While an EMS device may be able to temporarily strengthen, tone or firm a muscle, no EMS devices have been cleared at this time for weight loss, girth reduction, or for obtaining "rock hard" abs. The FDA has received reports of shocks, burns, bruising, skin irritation, and pain associated with the use of some of these devices. There have been a few recent reports of interference with implanted devices such as pacemakers and defibrillators. Some injuries required hospital treatment. Using these devices alone will not give you "six-pack" abs. Stimulating muscles repeatedly with electricity may eventually result in muscles that are strengthened and toned to some extent but will not, based on currently available data, create a major change in your appearance without the addition of weight loss and regular exercise.*[8]

Enough said. If you bought one of these devices, I know a way you could scare a certain post-operative patient in Augusta.

Another device that seems to rise from the ashes every few years is the infamous body wrap. You've seen the advertisements; just wrap this rubber sheet around your forty-inch waist and miracle of miracles, minutes later you have a twenty-eight-inch waist! Let me say that *any* claim that a device or cream targets spot reductions is false. Physiologically the body does not selectively lose weight from a particular area simply because you target it with a device or cream. You may tone a particular muscle group, but doing five thousand crunches will not remove fat exclusively from the abdominals. That's just not how it works.

Energy expenditure, age, and genetics dictate which and when fat deposits leave. So wrapping yourself in rubber may appeal to your spouse (that's another topic), but it will not "shrink away" or "dissolve" the pounds. The office of the Attorney General in Florida, who has prosecuted many fraud cases involving medical devices, reports, "Body wraps, cellulite creams, massages and other such quick 'fat reducers' are only temporary measures, at best, and have no long term effects on body fat."[9] In all fairness, these wraps do make you sweat, so if you are looking for a smelly, wet, ineffective tool for weight control, this is your item.

TIP-OFFS TO RIP-OFFS

The FDA has taken the lead on weeding out fraudulent practices in the weight loss and fitness world. This is a national problem because of the size of the industry and the billions of dollars spent. In an edition of their consumer magazine they compiled a list of "tip-offs to rip-offs," which are excellent statements to look for in any device being advertised to promote weight loss. Simply seeing these words in an advertisement doesn't necessarily mean it is a bad product; it just encourages you to thoroughly evaluate it for proof it accomplishes what it claims. (I couldn't resist embellishing their recommendations.)

🕺 *"This is safe and all natural."* Natural is the favorite buzzword of the slick marketers of our age. It is very similar to "Lite" of yesteryear. Remember when everything was referred to as lite: lite ice cream, lite chips, lite bulbs? However, no one really knew what lite meant until the government stepped in and demanded that anything bearing the moniker *lite* must meet certain requirements. That crown has now fallen to *natural.* No one knows what it means. In spite of this confusion (actually, maybe because of it), every product imaginable is labeled as natural, and it means nothing. The beer companies are especially savvy. They have a Natural Lite!

🕺 *"This revolutionary revelation is formulated by using proven principles of natural health based upon two hundred years of medical science."* It may be two hundred years of bad science; they don't say. This type of claim is wrought with errors, yet it remains popular to sell products. Words like *revolutionary* and *revelation* have connotations that imply success and authority—a classic marketing ploy.

🚶 *"Hunger stimulation point or thermogenesis, which converts stored fat into soluble lipids."* Watch out for meaningless medical jargon. It is incumbent on you to be aware of what is frivolous talk and what are reasonable claims. When an ad uses such language, it is for a purpose. Most advertisers target their ads to a fourth- or fifth-grade reading level. Their mantra is to keep it simple and direct. When you start seeing four- and five-syllable words, beware. They are most likely there only to impress and deceive. Any medical or nutritional concept can be explained in relatively simple language.

🚶 *"Lose 5 pounds a day."* Five pounds of what? Outrageous claims are usually just that . . . outrageous. If you take enough Ex-Lax you can lose five pounds in a day, but is that healthy? Remember, as a general rule, rapid weight loss is mostly water and will re-accumulate as fast as it is lost.[10]

The message is thunderously clear. There are no miracle machines, devices, or shortcuts . . . period! The sooner you acknowledge this, the quicker you are on your way to a fatter bank account instead of a fatter belly.

TAKE A PILL

Last week in my medical practice, I counted eight new requests for weight loss pills. It seems as if there is a pill for every malady, every shortcoming, every vice, or every illness facing us. The search for the perfect fat-busting pill has taken on somewhat of the aura of the quest for the Holy Grail, except that the grail in this case is a golden goose. The pharmaceutical companies realize that an effective, safe weight loss pill would be a blockbuster to end all blockbusters. It would catapult any company to the stratosphere of earnings, so needless to say, it is being actively pursued. The bad news for you venture capitalists is that it seems to be a long way off from arriving in our medicine cabinets (if ever). Although prescription medicines are not as shady as some "potions," I feel compelled to discuss them because there are elements of their marketing and use that should raise concerns. Some of these medicines are very useful;

however, many are abused and dangerous.

Prescription medicines for weight loss can be divided into two categories: appetite suppressants and fat-absorption blockers.

APPETITE SUPPRESSANTS

Appetite suppressants include such brand-name pills as Didrex, Tenuate, Sanorex, Mazanor, Adipex-P, Meridia, Bontril, and Ionamin. The infamous Phen-fen combination pill (phentermine and fenfluramine), which was pulled from the market in 1997, was also a member of this family. It should be noted that phentermine by itself is still available by prescription. Appetite suppressants promote weight loss by fooling the body into believing that it is not hungry. (Watching *Fear Factor* has the same effect!) They decrease appetite by increasing serotonin or catecholamine—two brain chemicals that affect mood and appetite. Most are amphetamines or amphetamine-like medications.

The most important fact to acknowledge about appetite suppressants is that they are designed for TEMPORARY use. If they are only safe—and there are those who even question that—for a few weeks to months, what happens in the ensuing decades in which you don't take them? I'll tell you (I like to provide help on these tough ones): you gain weight! I have heard the lame rationalization hundreds of times. "Doc, I just need something to get me going." Baloney! Be honest. What you want is a quick fix. It wouldn't be so bad if there weren't serious potential side effects of the medicines. These include potential addiction, increased heart rate, increased blood pressure, sweating, constipation, insomnia, excessive thirst, lightheadedness, drowsiness, stuffy nose, headache, anxiety, and dry mouth. Now *there's* a list you can wrap your belly around.

> "Diet pills are not recommended for use by teenagers because they are still growing, and if they suppress their appetite, they may not get proper nutrition. This is especially true of teenagers who don't need to lose weight but think that they do."
>
> —Michael Weintraub, MD, director of FDA's Office of Drug Evaluation

According to the American Society of Bariatric Physicians, the only people who should even consider these medicines are those that have a body mass index (BMI) of 30 and above with no obesity-related conditions, or a person with a BMI of 27 and above with obesity-related conditions (hypertension, diabetes, etc.). My own bias is that only very specific patients should ever resort to using these medicines, and then only under the care of a physician specially trained (ideally board-certified) in bariatric medicine.

For those looking to lose ten or twenty pounds, I see medications as a Band-Aid on a gaping wound. Those folks need a broader treatment plan that focuses on long-term lifestyle changes. In most incidences, medications are not suitable for children and teens.

FAT BLOCKERS

The second category of weight loss medicines is fat blockers. An example of this is orlistat (Xenical). Fat-absorption inhibitors work by preventing your body from breaking down and absorbing fat eaten with your meals. This unabsorbed fat is eliminated in bowel movements. This can result in diarrhea if fatty foods are consumed.

When I was a medical student, I was assigned to help in the care of Mrs. Slocum, a sweet sixty-eight-year-old lady who had a gastrointestinal problem that prevented her from absorbing proper nutrients. One of the foodstuffs that ran right through her was fat. She sticks in my mind because she is the only patient that I remember taking care of that I never saw outside of the bathroom. She was in the hospital for two weeks, and every time I came to see her, she was on the toilet. This was my introduction to poor fat absorption.

Taking these medicines certainly won't put you into the same state as Mrs. Slocum, but they can cause diarrhea if you eat fatty meals. In fact, one of the reasons for their success is that they discourage the eating of fatty foods to avoid the explosions that follow. This is somewhat like the aversion therapy I mentioned in an earlier chapter in that it changes your behavior by teaching you to avoid unpleasant consequences. I actually think these medicines can play a role in those who are very obese and trying to lose weight, because they don't just alter physiology, they also alter behavior. If the aversion to excessive dietary fat becomes imprinted, the benefits may last long after the medicine is stopped.

Some side effects with the fat blockers include abdominal cramping, passing gas, leakage of oily stool, increased number of bowel movements, and the inability to control bowel movements. These side effects are generally mild and temporary, but may be worsened by eating foods that are high in fat. Patients should start and maintain a low-fat diet (less than 30 percent of calories from fat) before starting treatment with these medicines. Because fat blockers reduce the absorption of some vitamins, you should take a multivitamin at least two hours before or after taking the medication.

Did You Know?

Ninety to 95 percent of people who lose weight with diet gain most of the weight back within three to five years. Oftentimes more body fat, or weight, is gained back.

Source: American College of Sports Medicine

Meridia and Xenical are the only weight loss medications approved for longer-term use in significantly obese people, although the safety and effectiveness have not been established for use beyond two years.[11]

Never take any weight control medicines without a thorough physical exam and proper monitoring. They are designed for a very select group of people, and for only a very short period of time.

SHOW ME THE MONEY

While studies are required to show that prescription medicines are relatively safe and effective before they come on the market, no such screening exists for herbs, plant substances, and vitamins. In a market where millions of dollars change hands every day, you must be skeptical and a very critical consumer. Every few months a new "wonder herb from the Amazon" or some other exotic sounding place is shouted from late-night infomercials. In one study, the Federal Trade Commission (FTC) investigated three hundred advertisements for 218 different weight loss products. The results were more than a little disturbing. "Nearly 40 percent of the ads in the study, including ads that appeared in mainstream, national publications, made at least one representation that is almost certainly false and 55 percent of the ads made at least one representation that is very likely to be false."[12]

CAUTION: CATCHPHRASES AHEAD

Accept the reality that when you purchase the latest herbal fad, you are chasing hot air and throwing dollars down to blanket your path! Save your money, time, and sanity, and avoid these scams. Here are some statements to look for by the most egregious offenders.

"Boost your metabolism and burn calories while you sleep." Many products that claim some special ability to do the miraculous are based on the substance ephedra or its derivative. This is a caffeine-like substance that has some properties similar to amphetamines. It was banned from use in dietary supplements by the FDA in 2004 because of a series of nasty side effects such as high blood pressure, irregular heartbeat, insomnia, nervousness, tremors, seizures, heart attacks, strokes, and even death. The problem is that some older ephedra-based products (before the ban) may still be around. Be sure you check ingredients in anything you propose to ingest. Be aware that substances such as the herbs Ma huang and guarana also have stimulant properties and can produce similar side effects. These products are still on the market and are in many weight control products. None have been shown to be consistently effective in the majority of people.

"Never feel hungry." The latest craze is the hoodia plant and its extracts used as an appetite suppressant. Hoodia is a cactus that is native to the Kalahari Desert in Africa. Natives supposedly eat it to reduce hunger during long hunts. This led to recent interest in it as a possible weight loss aid. One small study—sponsored by a supplement manufacturer—found that hoodia may affect the part of the brain that controls hunger. But much more research is needed to establish the potential effectiveness and long-term benefits and side effects. The Mayo Clinic newsletter recently stated, "There is no conclusive evidence that hoodia is an effective appetite suppressant."[13]

"Eat anything and block the fat." Chitosan has been touted as the ultimate fat binder that allows you to eat any fatty meal and not gain weight because the eager little chitosan molecules gobble up all the bad fat. Too good to be true? You bet it is! Chitosan is a fiber

supplement derived from the shells of crustaceans, which was shown to bind some fat in animal studies. Apparently this was all that the marketers needed to make claims that this substance would do the same in humans; however, they had nothing to back up that assumption. In fact, a study done by Dr. Judy Stern at the University of California-Davis showed that chitosan had no ability to bind fat and excrete it from the body.[14]

"Drink soothing herbal tea and lose the pounds." Herbal diet tea sounds harmless, but in fact it often contains potent laxatives, diuretics, or other drugs that can cause abdominal cramps, nausea, fainting, breathing difficulties, fluctuation in body temperature, and diarrhea. In addition . . . they don't work! Most act only as a purging laxative that temporarily reduces the fluid balance of the body. Many herbal diet teas on the market are unregulated and non-standardized as to ingredients or potency. This illustrates a bigger problem in that there is very little regulation of these "natural" products as to content and efficacy. Both the Federal Trade Commission and the Food and Drug Administration play a role in prosecuting false and potentially harmful products, but the volume of complaints is so high that the system naturally proceeds at a painfully slow pace. Regular teas, such as green tea, do have other health benefits and can be safely consumed.

"Amazing skin patch melts away body fat." In 2004 the FTC successfully sued a weight loss patch manufacturer for false and misleading claims about their product. According to the FTC, "This action targets a company that manufactured both an ineffective product and the misleading claims to sell it."[15] The patch people are guilty of a double deception in that they are placing substances in the patches that are unproven for weight loss, and there is little data to indicate that these substances are even absorbed into the body through the skin.

These are just a few of the examples of various herbs and substances that are on the market. Just like the weather, wait a few days and it will be different. Don't waste your time and money on diets and gimmicks. Don't jeopardize your family's health by teaching them to believe in these scams. Follow the commonsense guidelines of healthy balanced diets and exercise, and use all the money you save to take the family on an adventure vacation to Tahiti!

—— FAT-PROOF POINTERS ——

In dealing with scam diets, bogus nutritional supplements, and unhealthy practices, knowledge is power.

The tendency is for us to believe that we failed the diet rather than the other way around.

True hope lies in the only proven, long-term solution that has never been maligned or discounted: nutritionally balanced eating and smart exercise.

Seek independent resources for honest critiques of weight loss products or services.

There is no magic bullet, no holy grail of weight loss.

Diets don't work over the long term.

The low-carb craze excludes many known healthy foods such as fruits, vegetables, and whole grains.

Energy expenditure, age, and genetics dictate which and when fat deposits leave.

Prescription medicines for weight loss can be divided into two categories: appetite suppressants and fat-absorption blockers.

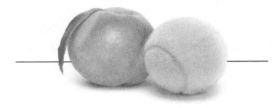

THE GOAL

ACHIEVING **WHOLENESS AND WELLNESS** AS A FAMILY

It's time to change our paradigms regarding health. We desperately need to shift our thinking from "me" to "us" when it comes to wellness. Everything we do, think, and feel impacts not only ourselves but also those who are a part of our world. This is especially true for those closest to us: our families. We must think of wellness not in terms of what I need to do or how I need to act, but how can both I and my family achieve wholeness. It bolsters your motivation and supplies the extra incentive needed to make radical changes. If you won't do it for yourself, do it for your family. So when you reread the previous chapters (and you know you should!) study them with the family in mind. We are a people of community, and it is through those communities that we define who we are and how we behave. No man or woman is an island, so what we think about our health and what we do about our wellness has a marked impact on those in community around us.

Not long ago, a lady came to my office telling a tale of woe that would make a statue cry. Her husband was fooling around on her, her son was in jail, her daughter was pregnant, her cat was hit by a car, and her dog had the mange! Her life was like a bad country song. After regaling for several minutes about her troubles, she stopped and abruptly said, "I'm so depressed . . . it must be my hormones!" I responded, "No, it's not; it's your life!" She was compartmentalizing things and not seeing the big picture. We can no longer afford to do that with our health.

The second change necessary is to view wellness from the perspective of the healing triad: mind, body, and spirit. Beginning in the 1980s, an increasing number of articles exploring the relationship between medicine and religion appeared in scientific journals. The writers brought about nothing less than a revolution in modern medical thinking as more and more physicians became aware of the vital role of thoughts, feelings, and emotions in the health of their patients. Works like Dale Matthews' *Faith Factors* and Harold Koenig's *Handbook of Religion and Health* once again reasserted the indelible relationship of the healing triad.

It is as if science and medicine now have come full circle from the ancients like Hippocrates who said it was not as important what kind of disease has the man as what kind of man has the disease. Dr. Herbert Benson, called the father of modern mind-body medicine, says, "Now, with many of the problems with drug therapy surfacing, people are looking to innate, inborn capabilities that are safe and effective. I think the future of health will be a three-legged stool where one leg is well-being, the other surgery, and the third self-care—and that is not only nutritional and not only exercise, but a major component is mind-body approaches and spirituality."[1] As Solomon wrote centuries ago, "A cheerful look brings joy to the heart; good news makes for good health" (Proverbs 15:30).

As we have seen, each component of the healing triad is independent yet intertwined with the other two as to create an inseparable identity. It is similar to the mobile that hangs over a child's crib. Each dangling object exists on its own, yet you can't touch one object without a response manifesting in the others. So it is with our health— our wholeness. If you spend all day weight lifting and building your muscles but spend no time developing relationships and your spiritual life, you end up being a very sad and lonely muscle-bound bore. Likewise, being a couch potato hampers the pursuit of emotional and spiritual health. Dr. James Gordon, professor of psychiatry and family medicine at Georgetown University, says, "It is time that we understand that the health of our minds and the health of our bodies are inextricably connected to the transformation of the spirit." [2]

THE MIRACULOUS BODY

You are a miraculous conglomeration of cells and chemicals. The awesome complexity and harmony of the physical body is almost unimaginable. The body contains between 10 and 100 trillion cells. These cells are in a constant cycle of breakdown, death, and remodeling. Every two to three days our intestines completely replace their lining cells, and our bones are turned over almost every seven years. We are constantly rebuilding even the most basic units of life. DNA, the blueprint for life that is present in every cell, illustrates the unbelievable complexity and perfect design of human beings. If you took the entire DNA in all the cells of the body and stretched it out end to end, it would reach for 2 million miles! Yet it can be compressed into the size of an ice cube.

Dr. Richard Swenson writes, "If after glimpsing the activity, intricacy, balance, and precision of life at this level you do not suspect a God standing behind it all, then my best diagnostic guess is that you are in a metaphysical coma."[3]

The more that is learned about the enormous precision and complexity of the physical functioning of the human, the more the evolutionists have to bow their heads and wonder. At the level of our understanding today, the Darwinist equation of *time + matter + chance = life* just looks foolish. John Herger writes in *Scientific American*, "Some scientists have argued that, given enough time, even apparently miraculous events become possible—such as this spontaneous emergence of a single-celled organism from random couplings of chemicals. Sir Fred Hoyle, the British astronomer, has said such an occurrence is about as likely as the assemblage of a 747 jet by a tornado whirling through a junkyard. Most researchers agree with Hoyle on this point."[4]

Yet even in the midst of this complexity and precision, the cell is still a cell, a heart a heart, and a brain a brain. They are tissues performing expertly their designated function, yet we still would not call all these tissues a human being without something more— something universal that ties it all together. There is a void that can only be filled by what theologians call the soul. It is what makes us human. It is the bridge between a collection of atoms and a creature created in the image of God. Our emotions can be reduced to a series of chemical changes, yet there is still the essence of the emotion, the *meaning* of the thought that defies physical explanation. That is what makes us human, different from other living creatures. We are God-breathed. Watchman Nee writes, "The spirit is that part by which we commune with God and by which alone we are able to apprehend and worship him."[5]

As our body is forever being remade, there is this spirit that remains constant, passed from one cell to the next. Without this essence, would our bones "remember" who we are if they are completely re-created every seven years? Would we have to re-learn our past experiences, feelings, or thoughts? The constant in this ever-changing body is the soul. This is our transcendent self that will live on after the physical body returns to the dirt from where it arose.

I believe the soul is separate from the mind. The mind represents the thoughts, feelings, and emotions that guide who we are and what we do. Again, as we learn more of neurophysiology, we can appreciate how feelings such as anger can be described in chemical terms. We know that certain areas in the brain, when stimulated by electrical currents, re-create emotions. Even aromas can cause memories locked deep in the cerebral tissue to be experienced as vividly as when they first occurred. The soul cannot be explained by equations or logic. It exists in the realm of transcendence—understood by God.

HEALING VS. CURING

I hope you are beginning to gain an appreciation that being fit is not just the absence of disease. Healing, in a biblical sense, is a balance between mind, body, and spirit. Curing is just simply ridding the body of the signs and symptoms of disease. Healing goes much deeper. Fat-proofing involves evaluating causes on all levels and proposes solutions that attempt to restore balance. Just as the ancients understood the concept of balance, we too have restructured our focus to embrace this concept.

I vividly remember the birth of my first daughter, Katie. At that point in my career, I had probably participated in over five hundred births. But this was different, so very different. People ask me if I delivered my children, and I laugh and say that I couldn't because my wife demanded she have a real doctor attend her! I couldn't agree with her more! But here I was seeing this little miracle emerge and take her first breath, and I was overwhelmed by the magnitude, the holiness, of what I was seeing. I had been very familiar with the mechanics of birth, yet I had truly not personally experienced the miracle of birth. It transformed me. From that point on I felt like a native instead of a tourist. I realized that the birth of this child was God's confirmation that the world was worth continuing.

Actually, that experience started me on a journey of spiritual exploration. Now, for the first time, I realized we were not just human beings in physical bodies, but spiritual beings in human bodies.

The biomechanical model of medicine is extremely limiting. The biblical concept of health not only expands the biomechanics of the body, but also incorporates the effects of the mind and spirit.

As a physician who is a Christian, I feel compelled to follow the path of healing outlined in the Bible. There is no disparity between science and Christian thought. I have stated before that all truth is of God. As Christians, we are not relegated to putting our minds on the shelf and ignoring the realities of the natural world. But we don't stop there either.

For example, if I truly believe in the healing power of prayer, then it is incumbent upon me to pray for and with my patients. Understand, this doesn't supplant my medical or surgical treatment; it compliments it. To some this may seem unusual and even unethical. However, I feel that Scripture is clear in stating that to deny this tool for healing is tantamount to spiritual malpractice. Without prayer, you are in danger of ignoring a vital part of a person's wellness, their spirit. Is this appropriate in every situation? Each person must answer that. Jesus didn't heal the same way in all cases. For some he touched, others he spoke words, and still others he called to action. In each case the underlying current was love. The *method* was not what healed; it was a loving compassion that opened the door for God's healing presence. So praying with a patient may be an essential part of the healing process in some instances, and in others it may not be what is needed at the time.

The Healing Triad

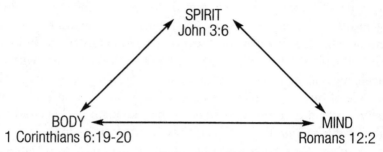

As you can see, all are dependent upon and affect the other. God, the source of healing, resides in the center, and each component of the healing triad draws strength from the others.

The concept of healing triad—mind, body, and spirit—is nicely summarized by Ebb Munden who said, "Germs do not cause disease. Germs are agents of disease, not the cause. Disease has its roots in an imbalance in our lives. Disease has its roots in the disintegration of the wholeness of our lives. This disintegration obstructs and blocks the natural healing energy that constantly seeks to flow through our lives. This disintegration of wholeness makes us vulnerable to disease to which we would not otherwise be susceptible."[6]

Fat-proofing your family is a calling that involves mind, body, and spirit. It is a choice . . . a tough choice. God provides the tools and resources, you provide the action. May your journey toward health and fitness be one of discovery and accomplishment.

> *Now may the God of peace make you holy in every way, and may your whole spirit and soul and body be kept blameless until that day when our Lord Jesus Christ comes again. God, who calls you, is faithful; he will do this.*
>
> *—1 Thessalonians 5:23–24*

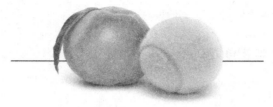

APPENDIX

EXERCISE TECHNIQUES

Before starting any exercise program, always have a good physical exam. Learn about any limitations dictated by your particular health needs, but more important, learn of your opportunities. Anyone, from a small child to a senior citizen, can learn these simple activities, but it may help to initially work with an exercise professional who will assist you in correctly using machines and weights if you choose that route. Even children and adolescents can use very light weights safely, and a certified trainer can design a safe regimen for those teens who want to progress. Many school athletic programs now have access to fitness experts who can work with teens and teach them proper and safe techniques.

Most of you new to exercise should begin slowly, using light weights and low intensity, and set goals for gradual improvement. Don't increase weight, intensity, or duration until your body adapts to the present activity, and that time frame can vary from person to person. In general, if you can comfortably do 12 repetitions at one weight, increase it by five pounds the next time. If you are able to walk twenty minutes without fatigue, either increase your speed or duration the next time out. Stay at that level until your body adapts, and then progress. Pick some activity that you enjoy, as this will improve your desire to follow through, and don't forget to encourage the whole family to participate.

BENCH PRESS (FOR THE CHEST)

While seated on the edge of a flat bench, grasp two dumbbells in an overhand grip.

Rest the dumbbells in an upright position on the edge of your knees. Carefully lie flat on the bench, bringing the dumbbells to the sides of your torso at chest level. Make sure to bring the dumbbells up simultaneously. Feet should be planted firmly on the floor.

Slowly press the weights up until your arms are fully extended. They will be at right angles to the floor. The dumbbells should be held directly over your chest area, slightly touching each other with palms facing forward.

EXECUTION

Slowly bend your elbows and lower both dumbbells in a slow, controlled fashion to your chest. The dumbbells should be at the sides of your chest.

Slowly press the weight back up from the sides of your chest to the starting position. Do not bounce the weight from the chest. Keep your elbows out and away from the trunk of your body. Keep the movement fluid, slow, and controlled.

SEATED ALTERNATE DUMBBELL CURLS (FOR THE BICEPS)

Using a bench, sit with your back straight and feet firmly planted on the floor. Grab a pair of dumbbells using an underhand grip and hold the arms in a down position.

EXECUTION

Slowly curl one dumbbell up toward your shoulder, pause, and slowly lower it. As you lower the dumbbell, curl the other arm upward. Do not swing the dumbbells up with any added body motion.

Keep the movement fluid, slow, and controlled.

SEATED DUMBBELL PRESS (FOR THE SHOULDERS)

In a seated position (I recommend using a bench with back support for this exercise) and with your feet firmly planted on the floor, grasp a dumbbell in each hand.

Curl the weight up to the shoulder area. Hold the dumbbells at shoulder level. Keep your back straight and your head up.

Make sure you rotate your palms so they are facing forward.

EXECUTION

In a controlled fashion, press the dumbbells simultaneously upward to the overhead position. The dumbbells should lightly touch each other at the top position. Do not arch the back. Slowly lower the weight down and repeat the movement.

Keep the movement fluid, slow, and controlled.

SQUATS (FOR THE LEGS AND BUTTOCKS)

Take a dumbbell in each hand. Keep your back and head straight. Your feet should be spaced at shoulder width. If you cannot squat flat-footed, try placing a two-by-four block of wood under your heels to improve balance.

EXECUTION

In a controlled fashion, slowly squat down until your thighs are parallel to the floor. Remember not to bounce at the bottom of the movement.

Slowly straighten your legs and return to the start position. Keep your head level at all times.

Keep the movement fluid, slow, and controlled.

STANDING CALF RAISES (FOR THE CALVES)

Standing upright, place your toes on a 1- or 2-inch elevation. Ensure that you are on the balls of your feet at the edge of the elevation.

Depending on your experience, you may hold a dumbbell in each hand.

Slowly drop your heels as far as they can go.

EXECUTION

Rise up as high as possible on the balls of your toes without excessive knee bending.

Slowly lower your heels as far as possible. Do not bounce at the bottom of the movement. Repeat.

Keep the movement fluid, slow, and controlled.

ABDOMINAL CRUNCHES

Lie on the floor with your knees bent and feet flat on the floor.

Cross your arms over your chest.

Push the lower back into the floor. Inhale slightly more than usual and hold your breath as you lift the head, shoulders, and upper back off the floor.

Concentrate on curling your upper trunk as much as possible.

Exhale and slowly return to the start position. During the entire movement, the neck should be held straight with the eyes looking at the ceiling.

LATERAL RAISES (FOR THE BACK)

Find a bench or other support and bend next to it at a 90-degree angle. Place your left hand on the bench for support.

Grasp a dumbbell with the right hand and bring it up in a straight line parallel to your shoulder.

Gently lower it to the original position.

Repeat using your other hand.

ADDITIONAL RESOURCES

HERBS AND NUTRACEUTICALS

Colbin, Annemarie. *Food and Healing*. New York: Ballantine Books, 1986.

Dorian, Terry. *Health Begins in Him*. Lafayette, La.: Huntington House, 1995.

Fugh-Berman, Adriane. *Alternative Medicine*. Baltimore: Williams and Wilkins, 1997.

Gazella, Karolyn. *Professional's Guide to Natural Healing*. Green Bay, Wis.: Impakt Communications, 1997.

Gladstar, Rosemary. *Herbal Healing for Women*. New York: Simon and Schuster, 1993.

Jensen, Bernard. *Foods That Heal*. Garden City, N.Y.: Avery, 1993.

Murray, Michael, and Joseph Pizzorno. *Encyclopedia of Natural Medicine*. Rocklin, Calif.: Prima Health, 1998.

PDR for Herbal Medicines. Montvale, N.J.: Medical Economics Company, 1998.

Vogel, H. C. A. *The Nature Doctor*. New Canaan, Conn.: Keats Publishing, 1991.

PRAYER

Breathnach, Sarah. *Simple Abundance*. New York: Warner Books, 1995.

Dossey, Larry. *Healing Words*. New York: HarperSanFrancisco, 1994.

Dossey, Larry. *Prayer Is Good Medicine*. New York: HarperSanFrancisco, 1997.

Foster, Richard. *Prayer: Finding the Heart's True Home*. New York: HarperSanFrancisco, 1992.

God's Little Devotional Book II. Tulsa, Okla.: Honor Books, 1997.

Koenig, Harold G. *The Healing Power of Faith*. New York: Simon and Schuster, 1999.

Owings, Timothy. *Hearing God in a Noisy World*. Macon, Ga.: Smyth and Helwys Publishing, 1998.

HUMOR

Adams, Patch. *House Calls*. San Francisco: Robert Reed Publishers, 1998.

Johnson, Barbara. *Living Somewhere Between Estrogen and Death*. Dallas: Word Publishing, 1997.

Klein, Allen. *The Healing Power of Humor*. Los Angeles: Jeremy Tarcher, 1989.

Samra, Cal, and Rose Samra. *More Holy Humor*. Nashville: Thomas Nelson, 1997.

EXERCISE

Bailey, Covert. *Smart Exercise*. New York: Houghton Mifflin, 1994.

NUTRITION

Bailey, Covert. *The New Fit or Fat*. New York: Houghton Mifflin, 1991.

Bailey, Covert. *The Fit or Fat Woman*. New York: Houghton Mifflin, 1989.

Baldinger, K. O. *Health and Nutrition*. Lancaster, Pa: Starburst, 1999.

Diamond, Harvey. *Living Health*. New York: Warner Books, 1987.

Goldberg, Albert. *Feed Your Child Right*. New York: M. Evans and Company, 2000.

Halliday, Arthur. *Thin Again*. Grand Rapids, Mich.: Revell, 1994.

McClure, Ed, and Elisa McClure. *Eat Your Way to a Healthy Life*. Lake Mary, Fla.: Siloam, 2006.

McMillen, S. I. *None of These Diseases*. Grand Rapids, Mich.: Revell, 1984.

Russell, Rex. *What the Bible Says About Healthy Living*. Ventura, Calif.: Regal, 1996.

Schlosser, Eric. *Fast Food Nation*. New York: Houghton Mifflin, 2002.

Weil, Andrew. *Eating Well for Optimum Health*. New York: Knopf, 2000.

GENERAL INTEREST

Backus, William. *The Healing Power of a Christian Mind*. Minneapolis: Bethany House, 1996.

Borg, Marcus. *Meeting Jesus for the First Time*. New York: HarperSanFrancisco, 1984.

Canfield, Jack, et al. *Chicken Soup for the Christian Soul.* Deerfield Beach, Fla.: Health Communications, 1997.

Craichy, K. C. *Super Health.* Minneapolis: Bronze Bow Publishing, 2005.

Hager, W. David. *As Jesus Cared for Women.* Grand Rapids, Mich.: Revell, 1998.

Little, Paul. *Know Why You Believe.* Wheaton, Ill.: Victor Books, 1987.

McGinnis, Alan Loy, *The Balanced Life.* Minneapolis: Augsburg, 1997.

Palms, Roger. *Bible Readings on Hope.* Minneapolis: World Wide Publications, 1995.

Remus, Harold. *Jesus as Healer.* New York: Cambridge Press, 1997.

Siegel, Bernie. *Prescriptions for Living.* New York: HarperCollins, 1998.

Sklare, John. The Inner Diet, *www.innerdiet.com.*

PARENTING

Cartmell, Todd. *The Parent Survival Guide.* Grand Rapids, Mich.: Zondervan, 2001.

Joslin, Karen. *Positive Parenting from A to Z.* New York: Ballantine Books, 1994.

Rosemond, John. *Parent Power.* Kansas City: Andrews and McMeel, 1990.

Rosemond, John. *Because I Said So.* Kansas City: Andrews and McMeel, 1996.

Schmitt, Barton. *Your Child's Health.* New York: Bantam, 1991.

NOTES

THE PROBLEM

1. A. A. Hedley, et al., "Prevalence of Overweight and Obesity Among U.S. Children, Adolescents, and Adults, 1999–2002." *Journal of American Medical Association* 291 (2004): 2847–50.
2. Jeffrey Ross, MD, "Obesity in Children," *American Medical Athletic Association Journal* (Spring 2006): 14.
3. Eric Schlosser, *Fast Food Nation* (New York: Houghton Mifflin, 2002), 4.
4. John Brant, "Team Hoyt," adapted from *Runner's World*, April 2006, 46.
5. *Runner's World*, April 2006.

A BEGINNING

1. *www.innerdiet.com.*
2. Ann Kelley, "Opioid-Mediated Binge Eating of Fat," *NeuroReport*, August 2004.
3. Andrew Weil, *Eating Well for Optimum Health* (New York: Alfred A. Knopf, 2000), 12.
4. Schlosser, *Fast Food Nation*, 5.
5. Ibid., 5.
6. Ibid., 4.
7. Kimberly Truesdale and J. Stevens, "Do the Obese Know They Are Obese?" *Experimental Biology Journal* 20 (March 7, 2006).
8. E. Kyung and J. C. Rhee, "Parenting Styles and Overweight Status in First Grade," *Pediatrics* 117 (2006): 2047–54.

9. Adapted from David Elkind, *The Hurried Child* (New York: Addison-Wesley, 1988), 84.
10. C. S. Lewis, *The Abolition of Man* (New York: McMillan Publishing, 1962), 78.

THE PARENTAL MANDATE

1. John Rosemond, *Because I Said So* (Kansas City: Andrews and McMeel, 1996), 25.
2. Brenda Jank, "Once a Gift, Now a Treasure," Focus on the Family, 2004, *www.family.org.*
3. Elena Poveda, "Association Between Anxiety and Depressive Disorders in Adolescents and Family Meals," *Journal of Epidemiology and Community Health* 56 (2002): 89–94.
4. "Family Dinner Linked to Better Grades for Teens," April 2005, *www.ABCnews.com.*
5. Jennifer Yates, "Hospital Offers Obesity Program for Kids," April 27, 2006. *www.washingtonpost.com.*
6. J. C. Eisenmann, et al., "Relationship Between Adolescent Fitness and Fatness and Cardiovascular Disease Risk Factors in Adulthood," *American Heart Journal* 149, no.1 (January 2005): 46–53.

NUTRITION BASICS

1. Alok Bhargava, "The Women's Health Trial Feasibility Study of Minority Populations," *British Journal of Nutrition* (December, 2002).
2. Weil, *Eating Well for Optimum Health,* 6.
3. R. L. Weinsier, "Medical-Nutrition Education: Factors Important for Developing a Successful Program," *American Journal of Clinical Nutrition* 62 (1995): 837.
4. David Barboza, "If You Pitch It, They Will Eat" (*New York Times,* August 3, 2003).
5. T. Colin Campbell, *The China Study* (Dallas: Benbella Books, 2004), 2.
6. Ibid., 88.
7. D. S. Ludwig, "Dietary Glycemic Index and the Regulation of Body Weight," *Lipids* 38, no. 2 (2003):117–121.
8. L. E. Spieth, et al., "A Low-Glycemic Index Diet in the Treatment of Pediatric Obesity," *Archives of Pediatric and Adolescent Medicine* 154, no. 9 (2000): 947–951.
9. D. Y. Jones, "Influence of Dietary Fat on Self Reported Menstrual Symptoms," *Physiology and Behavior* 40 (1987): 483–7.

10. C. Longcope, "The Effect of a Low Fat Diet on Estrogen Metabolism," *Journal of Clinical Endocrinology and Metabolism* 64 (1987):1246–50.
11. R. Norris and C. Sullivan, *PMS* (New York: Berkley Publishing, 1983), 64.
12. R. Russell, *What the Bible Says About Healthy Living* (Ventura, Calif.: Regal Books, 1996), 27.
13. Weil, *Eating Well for Optimum Health,* 204.

FOOD FOR THE SOUL

1. Campbell, *The China Study,* 10.
2. S. I. McMillen, *None of These Diseases* (Grand Rapids: Revell, 1984), 84.
3. "The New Testament," an audio series from The Teaching Company, 2006.

CHILDREN AND TEENS

1. U.S. Food and Drug Administration, "Food Allergies Rare but Risky," December 2004, *www.cfsan.fda.gov.*
2. Albert Goldberg, *Feed Your Child Right* (New York: M. Evans and Co., 2000), 99.
3. Schlosser, *Fast Food Nation,* 52.
4. Ibid, 56.
5. Goldberg, *Feed Your Child Right,* 83.

WEIGHT LOSS

1. Campbell, *The China Study,* 140.
2. Associated Press, "Food for Thought," *Atlanta Journal Constitution,* January 3, 2005.
3. Jeffrey Friedman, "A War on Obesity, Not the Obese," *Science,* February 2003, 857.
4. Weil, *Eating Well for Optimum Health,* 98.
5. Joel Fuhrman, *Fasting and Eating for Health* (New York: St. Martins, 1995), 184.
6. T. D. Jakes, *Lay Aside the Weight* (Minneapolis: Bethany House, 2002), 52.

EXERCISE

1. Jay Stoll, "A Comparison of Exercise and SSRI Medications on Mild Depression" *Archives of Internal Medicine* 159, no. 19 (1999):2349–56.

2. Alice Feinstein, ed., *Training the Body to Cure Itself* (Emmaus, Pa.: Rodale Press, 1992), 3.
3. Ibid, 7.
4. "Sedentary Children," *UC-Davis Health Journal* (September 2000).
5. Dirk Johnson, "Many Schools Putting an End to Child's Play," *New York Times*, April 7, 1998, A1, A16.
6. David Ross, "Type II Diabetes and Mortality," *American Medical Athletic Association Journal* (Winter 2006): 14.
7. H. G. Koenig, *The Healing Power of Faith* (New York: Simon and Schuster, 1999), 100.
8. American College of Obstetricians and Gynecologists Clinical Opinion, 2004.

BEWARE

1. L. Fraser, *Losing It* (New York: Dutton, 2001), 47.
2. Tracie Johanson, "Why Diets Don't Work," *www.stanford.edu*, April 2004.
3. "Weighing the Evidence in Diet Ads," Federal Trade Commission, November 2004, *www.ftc.gov*.
4. Carol Foster, "A Weighty Problem," University of Michigan health systems, Feb 2003, *www.med.umich.edu*.
5. *Journal of the American College of Nutrition* 22 (2003): 9.
6. M. L. Dansinger, et al., "One Year Effectiveness of the Atkins, Ornish, Weight Watchers, and Zone Diets in Decreasing Body Weight and Heart Disease Risk," presented at the American Heart Association Scientific Sessions, November 12, 2003 in Orlando, Florida; *New England Journal of Medicine* 348 (2003):2082; *Annals of Internal Medicine* 140 (2004): 778, 523; *Preventive Cardiology* 5 (2002): 110.
7. Heidi Michels Blanck, et al., "Use of Low-Carbohydrate, High-Protein Diets Among Americans," Centers for Disease Control, 2005.
8. "Six-Pack Abs Electronically?" *FDA Consumer magazine,* July-August 2002.
9. "How to Protect Yourself from Health Fraud," *www.myfloridalegal.com*, 2007.
10. Paula Kurtzweil, *FDA Consumer magazine,* November-December 1999, (comments my own).
11. "WIN Notes," National Institute of Diabetes, Digestive and Kidney Disease, *www.win.niddk.nih.gov,* 2003.
12. Federal Trade Commission, "Report on Weight-Loss Advertising," *www.ftc.gov/opa/2002/09/weightlossrpt.htm*.

13. Jennifer Nelson, "Is Hoodia an Effective Appetite Suppressive?" *www.MayoClinic.com,* 2005.
14. M. D. Gades and J. S. Stern, "Chitosan Supplementation Does Not Affect Fat Absorption in Healthy Males Fed a High-Fat Diet," *International Journal of Obesity and Related Metabolic Disorders* 26 (2002):119–122.
15. "Skin Patches Don't Cause Weight Loss," Federal Trade Commission, *www.ftc.gov.* 2004.

THE GOAL

1. Testimony before the U.S. House of Representatives, *Journal of the American Psychological Association* (November 1997).
2. Daniel Redwood, "Manifesto for a New Medicine," *www.healthy.net,* 2006.
3. R. Swenson, *More than Meets the Eye* (Colorado Springs: Navpress, 2000), 21.
4. Ibid., 191.
5. Watchman Nee, *The Spiritual Man* (Richmond, Va.: Christian Fellowship Publishers,1977), 27.
6. J. Wagoner, *An Adventure in Healing and Wholeness* (Nashville: Upper Room Books, 1993), 21.